COMPLEXION, COSMETICS, AND THE CHRISTIAN

(Formally "Ashamed of my Color")

By
Dr. Ebenezer A. Nwankwo

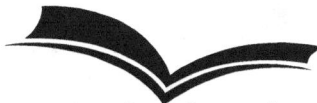

TEACH Services, Inc.

P U B L I S H I N G

www.TEACHServices.com • (800) 367-1844

Copyright © 2007, 2019 Ebebezer A. Nwankwo
Copyright © 2007, 2019 TEACH Services, Inc.
ISBN-13: 978-1-57258-466-2 (Paperback)
Library of Congress Control Number: 2007925770

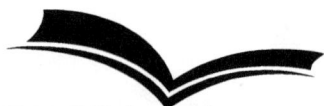

TEACH Services, Inc.
P U B L I S H I N G
www.TEACHServices.com • (800) 367-1844

Dedicated to Glory,
a wife and mother of exceptional character

TABLE OF CONTENTS

LIST OF DIAGRAMS

PREFACE

The issue of complexion, cosmetics and the Christian, which is the subject of this brief book, has been on the preachers' pulpit in the recent past. Views and perceptions of the use of cosmetics differ among the preachers. But all agree that moral beauty or character takes precedence over physical appearance and beauty.

A work on related issue of color prejudice focuses on racism from the view point of a historian. Otherwise, writers are few and unsystematic on the issue of complexion and application and use of makeup by Christians.

Conservative preachers objecting to the use of makeup argue that such use implies a denial and rejection of God's perfect and complete creation in man. This view, however, does not consider the result of sin and effects of diseases on human body that may require care and treatment with the use of some cosmetic preparation/drug. On the other hand, some liberal preachers, and beauty therapists encourage the use of makeup as a right to keep and maintain a decent physical appearance. Granted, but motivating factors for the use of makeup, much more involving than the makeup, are ignored. Besides, God's right to receive honor and glory from man cannot be replaced with man's right to a life-style of self-centeredness.

No objective discussion of the application and use of makeup by Christians apart from human complexion. The first step to understanding the significance of human complexion is to consider the source and reason for man's existence. Once we have established the source and place of human complexion, we can begin to examine the place of cosmetics in human existence. To illuminate this point is the *raison d'etre* of this brief book. I have tried in this book to consider, from creationist and biblical point of view, the dangers associated with preoccupation with outward appearance if and when moral character, the inner beauty is marginalized.

After all, no one argues against the fact that beauty of character, not makeup beauty, brings life-long joy and happiness, and leaves a happy memory from generation to generation.

The book examines the development of complexion, noting the inter-relatedness and organic bond of all the human skin colors. Also, examined is the history of the use of makeup and its cultural, emotional and sexual significance in our society. This, perhaps, makes the book a unique treatise on complexion and the use of cosmetics. Those familiar with my earlier book, Ashamed of my color, will find in *Complexion, Cosmetics and the Christian*, a thorough editing and revisions of all chapters, reflecting objective treatment of the issue.

—The Author

ACKNOWLEDGMENTS

Grateful acknowledgment is made to the following for permission to reprint copyrighted material:

Grolier Incorporated From "Cosmetics" by Letitia L. Sage from *The Encyclopedia Americana*, 2000 edition; From "Makeup" by Herman Buchman from *The Encyclopedia Americana*, 2000 edition.

Atlas Editions, Inc. From "Cosmetics" by Henry Goldschmeidt, Morris B. Jacobs and Ernest Kuehns from *Collier's Encyclopedia, vol.* 7. From "Skin Color" by Harold Cummins from *Collier's Encyclopedia*, vol. 21

Prentice-Hall, Inc. From *The Human Venture: A World History from Prehistory to the present*. 3rd edition by Anthony Esler.

Keter Publishing House Ltd. From "Cosmetics in the Talmud" by Eli Davis from *Encyclopedia Judaica*, vol. 5.

I thank Dr. Abraham Kuranga, Ph.D. a first reader of the book, who offered some helpful suggestions and opinions that led to additional materials to clarify the issue, and Dr. Karen Kossie-Chernyshev of Texas Southern University who challenged me to think broader and deeper on historical issues of the "colored" and the "colorless."

INTRODUCTION

Many a lonely tomb across the nations of the world would have its epitaph read: "Died in search of physical beauty." Many a healthy man or woman has died from the complications of cosmetic surgery. The living becomes emotionally hurt by the loss. The tomb reminds the living the cost to or effect of a passion for external physical appearance upon the self and others. The effect of a lifestyle is ultimately an outcome of a choice prompted by a perception of the self and others. Conversely, a perception is translated into intra-personal and interpersonal relationships.

How is your intrapersonal relationship like? I mean your attitude and reaction to what you perceive, think and believe you are, and value placed upon the self. Do you know how one relates to oneself is as important and critical as interpersonal relationship? By design, both intra-personal and interpersonal relationships generate in the mind. Interestingly, the work of the Psycho physiologist supports Biblical intimation of a correlation between the mind and behavior (Prov. 15:13-15; 17:22; 23:7; Luke 6:45). Our perception is reflected in our lifestyle, and our lifestyle affects us personally and other people around us. There is no doubt the mind has a controlling influence on our lifestyle. Further, how we live is a reflection of our attitude and values. Consequently, our attitude, the state of our mind or feeling, and our values affect our relationships. Perhaps, people do not see how intra-personal and inter-personal relationships are affected in every lifestyle, but effects of our lifestyle on both the self and other persons are apparent. Obviously, any lifestyle affects our intrapersonal and interpersonal relationships. The cosmetics lifestyle is no exception. It is sanctimonious, however, to regard cosmetics lifestyle as a matter of right or wrong-suggesting the use of cosmetics immoral, and non-use of cosmetics moral. The suggestion is as judgmental as taking the place of God in his judgment seat.

The issue of cosmetics and human complexions is, basically, a question of the essence of human existence, namely, individuality, freedom, and responsibility. These three elements are collectively an attribute of a moral being. As a way of clarity, individuality is expressed in freedom to think and act independently. Freedom is a right to choose and act responsibly. Responsibility is a burden of care, an account for result or effect of one's choice and action. Unfortunately, some consider the essence of human existence in defense of their preoccupation to outward appearance and beauty. The use of cosmetics is defended as a personal matter and any body's right. Granted, but the effect and implications of cosmetics are never ever thought of or considered by the defense. The fact of the matter is that one has the right to independently choose and act on one's choice. But every choice we make reflects our perception of the world in relation to the self and other people. Therefore, one is answerable for the effect of that choice. On the other hand, our perceptive differences explain why we respond differently to a common situation. For example, in a struggle between how we look and what we think we ought to be like, some would settle for "improving" their physical form and complexion. They would turn to cosmetics to create a "new self" and look like their dream figure. Some take to cosmetic surgery, altering their natural physical build. Some turn to skin lighteners and other makeup preparations, and still some chose to tan their skin.

Undoubtedly, we have one time or the other felt dissatisfied with the way we look. But why do so many Christians and non-Christians adopt cosmetics lifestyle, at a time when the world needs quality moral character, the inner beauty for the ills of the heart? The universal adoption of the style, its appeal to every sex and age is a social trend, glorifying comely body and outward appearance. Therefore, there is no better time than now to evaluate the place of cosmetics and human complexion in light of the overall purpose and meaning of life. Also a twin problem of discontent and aversion to human complexion is considered in reference to our existence in relationships.

A typical example of an aversive attitude toward human skin color is illustrated in the story of two pen pals, Bokee and Poku.

The two pals lived two worlds apart with cultural and religious differences. They pen palled for years and never saw or exchanged their photos with each other. However, after a couple of years they agreed to meet at a certain place and on a certain day and time. When Bokee, with his puppy, Ure, arrived at the meeting place, he was glad to meet with Poku who had arrived a few minutes earlier. After a brief introduction, Bokee offered a handshake but received a cold response from Poku. However, Poku reached out for Ure and carried the puppy in his arms. Poku spoke of his admiration for Ure. Bokee could not understand the cold response. He looked at Poku and asked, "Were you expecting me or a dog?" "I am sorry," Poku, replied, "I was not expecting a colored person." "Why," Bokee asked. Poku was blunt, "you know, Mr. Bokee, a mismatch of colors or anything does not make for a pleasant site or harmony. I am not going to be mismatched either." Bokee was disappointed with the answer. When he inquired further why Poku tolerated and admired the puppy whose hair color is similar to Bokee's skin color. Poku responded, "I admire Ure for what it is, a dog, and not its look or hair color. "Besides, he continued, "Do you not know that a dog is every man's best friend?" Poku's ethnocentric bias is evident. As a matter of opinion, Poku represents the thinking and value system of the "colorless" that feels uncomfortable working and associating with the "colorful." It is not unnatural with man to feel threatened or suspicious of unfamiliar person.

But why should one prefer a non-human for friendship to a fellow human? Why should one tolerate a dog for what it is, but not willing to accept one's fellows for who they are in spite of their complexion?

Every Christian should be mentally and morally challenged by the problems and questions raised by the different situations described.

We shall address the problems from the historical and biblical perspectives. A review of the factors that impact the problems, the ethical and theological implications of the remedial approach to the problems are made in reference to Christians. Because of their claim to a divinely inspired book, the Bible, that prescribes a standard of conduct for all. Also the Christians believe in Jesus, the divine author of the Bible who taught them how to live. The study is prompted by two considerations, first, the case of Limah who symbolically gave up her natural and colorful identity to fit in with the crowd, and second, the attitude of some men and women who with ethnic considerations consider their fellows second class citizens in a world of God's making. Still some professed Christians who cannot tolerate seeing their fellows live and move freely in the social, economic, and political world of man's making.

Chapter 1

LIMAH AND HER MAKEUP

An Eye witness Account:

Limah was twenty-four years old and the mother of two beautiful girls. The recent death of her parents and a lover has forced on her the burden of caring for the kids. In a town whose population was divided on racial lines, and where a few influential and powerful politicians controlled the economy, job openings were rare and competitive for a high school dropout like Limah. Besides, her skin color, accent, and family background posed an obstacle to her full integration into the social and economic life of the town. Lack of job skill was a source of frustration too. She performed odd jobs, and lived from hand-to-mouth existence.

Limah's acquaintance with Remo, a friend of a wealthy grocery store owner, landed her a job as a sales assistant in a small local grocery store. For a couple of months, Limah dressed well and simply at work. Each working day she would feel out of fashion with her co-workers and customers. Soon Limah began to use bleaching soap and creams for a lighter skin. She was also hooked into wearing some makeup on her lips and nails.

One early morning, when Limah was putting on her makeup and getting ready for work, her six year old daughter came to her and asked, "Mom are you going to act a play at the theater?" Limah looked at her daughter and said, "Honey, I am not going to theater. I am going to work at the grocery." Dissatisfied with her mother's answer, the little girl asked, "Is there a theater at the grocery store?" "Why, honey?" Limah retorted. "You are dressed like an actress, Mom," exclaimed the six-year old girl. Limah in a subdued tone responded, "You don't understand now, but you will in a few years' time.

1

The girl grew to tell of this encounter with her mother and how at one point she held back herself from asking, "Mom are you ashamed of your color"?

Is the little girl's observation an outburst of an inquisitive mind or an ignoramus?

Do you see it as an expression of innocence, and simplicity? Does the girl's observation offer any food for thought? Further, one is poised to ask: "Why would one think of changing or "improving" one's natural complexion? Is discontent with one's skin color a rejection of God's wisdom and magnanimous gift? Or is it to be dismissed as merely a personal choice and matter without consequences?

Well, this section is about makeup. The meaning of makeup and its use in history are briefly surveyed. The section focuses, first, on human skin color from the viewpoint of evolutionary theory, and the biblical account of creation; secondly, on the various reactions to human skin colors in our day and in the Bible times

What is Cosmetic?

The term "cosmetic" comes from the Greek word, *Kosmetikos* [skilled or competent in adornment]. Its verb form, *kosmein*, means to adorn or arrange in order. The term refers to preparation and /or material used for beautifying the human complexion.

There are a wide variety of preparations grouped together under the general term, "cosmetics". These preparations include: creams and lotions for cleansing and improving the appearance of the skin; manicure and makeup preparations for improving with colorings the nails and complexion; grooming and hair preparations.

Cosmetics, generally, are a preparation and man's device for enhancing the physical appearance of human body so as to look beautiful and attractive. In addition, actors and actresses wear these preparations and costumes to project the image of another character (see Letitia L. Sage. "Cosmetics", *The Encyclopedia Americana*, International edition, Vol. 8, Danbury, Connecticut: Grolier Inc., 2000, 33; cf. Herman

Buchman, "Makeup", ibid. Vol. 18, Danbury, CT: Grolier Inc., 2000, 149).

Cosmetic, in its implied usage, is a compensator, that which makes up or offsets a lack or want. If thus viewed and used, cosmetic is a human compensatory preparation for a perceived or imaginary lack or deficiency on the wearer's physical appearance and complexion.

Our discussion on cosmetics does not include the following preparations and procedures:

1. Fragrance products, such as perfumes or deodorants.

2. Therapeutic preparations which include lubricating or moisturizing creams, lotions and ointments for skin diseases, dry, flaking skins and/or chapped lips.

3. Plastic surgery. A surgical procedure for restoring or correcting disfigured limb or part of the body due to accident, disease or infection.

Also, not included in the discussion is the traditional African "tanjele" or "teero/tiro". This is a type of limestone, soft and bluish. The Arab merchants, probably, introduced it to the Sub-Saharan Africa some centuries before the colonial era. The soft bluish limestone is grinded into powdery form, slightly wetted, and rubbed on the eyelashes and eyelids. It is claimed to be therapeutic, worn to prevent and/or clear eye infection. This claim, however, is disputed on the ground that mostly women use "tanjele" or teero/tiro on special occasions.

The discussion is limited and exclusively to manicure and makeup preparations, complexion altering creams, and cosmetic plastic surgery.[1] Cosmetic surgery is included because of the author's conviction that any alteration of the size or shape of human body parts such as the nose, eye, or the breast in order to "improve" appearance or look attrac-

---

1   The nature of this class of cosmetic preparations, and procedure raises the issue discussed in this book. Their material contents work to correct, alter, and improve the authentic skin color and/or external features of the human body.

tive is godlessness. Besides, unlike plastic surgery, cosmetic surgery is not due to any accident, disease or infection of the tissues of the body parts. The choice for and objection to some cosmetic preparatoins may seem arbitrary. None-the-less, some skin diseases, dry, flaking skin, chapping lips, and etc., for example, would require the use of appropriate cosmetic/drug preparatoins for treatment.

Makeup in History

Makeup is not the creation or invention of modern times, but one of the practices of ancient peoples that has survived to this day, though it has been perfected and used in a much wider scope today than it was in ancient times. Among the ancient peoples that used makeup were the Egyptians. They used it for religious purposes, embalming their dead and painting the eyes of their idols. The Egyptians also used cosmetics for personal adornment (see Henry Goldschmeidt, Morris B. Jacobs and Ernest Kuehns, "Cosmetics", *Collier's Encyclopedia*, Vol.7, New York: Collier's, 1997, 363).

In the book of Esther we read about a national beauty contest for young women sponsored by a Persian king. The beauty parade gave the king an opportunity to choose a wife. Each contestant spent a full year with beauty treatments. The twelve month beauty regimen consisted of a prescribed body treatment with oil of myrrh, perfumes, body lotions and/or creams (Esther 2:3–12).[2] It appears from the narrative that the use of makeup was promoted by the state. The length of time for the beauty regimen afforded the judges an opportunity to watch closely and observe the contestants in a controlled harem environment. The Persian king with his counselors knew by personal experience that moral character is as important, if not more desirable, as external beauty. The king recently divorced Vashti, his wife, who is described as "lovely to look at" (Esther 1:10). The king needed someone morally better and virtuous than Vashti. A posted vacant position of a queen in the kingdom caught the attention of Mordecai who encouraged his adopted daughter, Esther to join

---

2   All Bible references in this work are from the New International Version (NIV), unless otherwise stated.

the contest. Esther was an orphan, raised in the modest and single home of her uncle. She is described as "lovely in form and features" (Esther 2:7). The Bible indicates, also, that all the beauty contestants were beautiful (Esther 2:2). But Esther had what other contestants lacked. She pleased and found favor with all that saw and met with her (Esther 2:9, 15, 17). Trusting in her natural physical beauty and the charm of her character, Esther needs no more than a simple cosmetic prepations, such as fragrance products, some grooming and non-bleaching body and hair lotions and creams. Esther's pleasant demeanor and posture made a difference. Her moral and physical beauty won for her the enviable crown and position (Esther 2:15, 16, 17).

It is reported that the Jewish Talmud approved of makeup for women. Every Jewish wife considered it a duty to beautify herself with some makeup. This is with the objective of appearing attractive to her husband (see Eli Davis, "Cosmetics in the Talmud", *Encyclopedia Judaica*, Vol. 5, Jerusalem: Keter Publishing, 1971, 980).

Some cultural groups in Africa, south of the Sahara, also used makeup. They extracted or prepared their makeup from the bark, roots, and fruits of some special plants and woods. The women wore makeup during festivals, annual or seasonal cultural dances and displays.

Historically, the use of makeup can be dated back to the Garden of Eden, in the Near East. Stretch your mind and eyes to the first theatrical scene and performance on earth. The lone actor was Lucifer. The one and only audience was Eve. The platform was the tree at the center of the Garden of Eden. There, Lucifer, the master actor, was projected in the image of another character, the Serpent. How could Lucifer do that? The Bible indicates: "Satan himself transforms himself into an angel of light" (2 Cor. 11:14, NKJV). Satan falsely assumed the appearance and the look of another character. Eve was captivated, enticed, and deceived by the physical appearance and mimic expressions of the Devil in the person of the Serpent.

The working principles and end results for the use of makeup today are similar to Lucifer's stratagem in the Garden of Eden. Satan's disguise in the Garden parallels today's actors' wearing makeup. The actors' aim for the use of makeup is different from Satan's goal for disguising himself. However, the projection of another person's image and the resultant deception are essential features common to Satan's disguise, and the use of makeup today.

A definition and brief survey of the use of makeup in history are used as a point of departure. The chapters that follow will discuss the human skin color and its origin from the viewpoint of the evolutionist, and from the biblical perspective. Reactions and problems associated with human complexion are also examined.

Cosmetics

The "makeup" body negates the Savior's homely body.
The eye shadow in contemn of the Savior's eye salve.
The lipstick tinted to stain parallels the vinegar-soaked
sponge tilted to the Savior's lips and pain.
The painted lips and adorned body a mockery of our
Savior's bruised lips and marred body.
Let the world see not your manicured nails and hands
but the Savior's nail-scarred hands.
The world's a stage, nay, a preparatory University for
a makeover life for Jesus here and hereafter.

Chapter 2

HUMAN SKIN COLOR

Evolution and Skin Color

Some scientist, genetic engineers, and historians currently theorize a common ancestry from East Africa, for the entire human race. The East African ancestor through whom all the human species evolved lived for many millennia in the present continent of Africa. The human beings who, probably, evolved from the "African Eve" migrated to various parts of the world. The wandering groups in search of food and, eventually, settled life encountered differing weather conditions. Consequently these migrant descendants of the African Eve developed over the ages skin pigments that helped them adapt to, and survive, through the climatic conditions found in their settled locations (see Anthony Elser, *The Human Venture: A World History from Prehistory to the Present*, 3rd edition, Upper Saddle River, NJ: Prentice Hall, 1996, 8, 10, 11).

From the viewpoint of the evolutionists, the varied skin colors of the human race today evolved with time. The skin colors evolved to meet the varied climatic conditions, which were encountered by the various groups of descendants of the African Eve. This view is in harmony with the strongly held concepts of evolutionary theory. The theory asserts that 1) organisms bear the characteristics of their progenitors; 2) the characteristics of these living things change with time; and 3) traits or hereditary makeup that are latent in the progenitors or parents may be visible in their descendants.

If we believe in the theory of the African origin of the human race, then the skin color of the African Eve cannot be disputed. Some of the descendants of the African Eve inherited the same skin color of their progenitor. Others developed skin pigments different from the skin color of their ancestor. The evolutionist may credit the different complexion to inherited traits or evolved structural adaptation to the climate.

In the light of the evolutionary theory and concept, we concluded that black was, probably, the skin color of the African Eve. All the other human skin colors were latent in her. The lighter skin pigment and the brown-yellow skin colors developed with her offspring with time to meet the changing weather conditions.

The theory of the African Eve offers a common ancestry for all humankind. It also attests for a common source of human skin colors. That common source or bearer is the African Eve.

The Bible and Skin Color

The Bible offers a somewhat detailed account of the origin of all living things. An introduction of the history of creation of all things begins with such expressions as "These are the generations of the heavens and the earth when they were created" (Gen. 2; 4, KJV). Also the history of the human family is introduced by the expression, "This is the generations of Adam" (Gen. 5:1), and "These are the generation of Noah" (Gen. 6:9, KJV). The genealogies in the book of Genesis and the gospel of Luke demonstrate a common ancestry for humankind. The biblical account of the creation claims Adam and Eve as the ancestors of human race (Gen. 1:27, 28; Gen. 2:18, 22). The account testifies further that Adam was of the dust of the ground. God, the divine potter, manipulated the dust/clay to form a living human being, (Gen. 2:7; cf. Isa. 64:8; Job 10:8, 9).

The soil layer of the Garden of Eden from which Adam was formed is essentially no different from the soil layers of the earth today. There was the dark soil, the red soil, and the brown-colored soil. Adam's skin color must in essence be similar to the color of dust/clay, "since from it (ground) you were taken; for dust you are, and to dust you will return" (Gen 3:19). Adam and Eve were, probably, of one and same skin color. They were, genetically, carriers of other skin pigments, which they passed on to their offspring.

The skin color of this Near Eastern couple may have been either brown[1] or yellow-brown. However, the biblical account has it that some descendants of these Near Eastern ancestors were black. For example, the second river Gihon from the Garden of Eden flowed to water the land of Cush, the dark-colored people of Ethiopia (Gen. 2:13).

God created the world to be inhabited (Isa. 45:18). He commanded Adam and Eve and their descendants to procreate and fill the earth (Gen. 1: 27, 28). God is aware of the various differing geographical and climatic conditions that would exist on the earth.

He clothed each group of the human race—Caucasoid, Mongoloid, Negroid, etc.—with skin color, which is unique with that group (Job 10:11). God designed and determined from the beginning the various skin pigments. He did not leave the color of the skin to be determined by weather or climate. Otherwise Adam and Eve were neither created with skin color nor perfectly and completely created. Skin color is an inextricable texture of the human body. It is what visibly differentiates, for example, the American Indian from the African American.

The Antediluvians were probably not of the same color. There was the black, the light, and the yellow-brown colored skin. These differing skin colors were not the result of inbreeding, and geographical or environmental conditions. Because the Antediluvians lived and enjoyed the same climatic conditions of their times. Similarly, the Postdiluvian were of varied skin colors. At a point in time, in the biblical history of the human race, the Postdiluvian spoke one common language (Gen. 11:1). They banded together to build themselves a tower that would house their residential and commercial needs and ventures. But such an attempt to congregate into one geographical location is a direct violation and disregard of God's plan to have the human race replenish the earth.

God acted swiftly to confuse their one common language. With the confusion of the common language, numerous languages were developed, thus forcing them to scatter and dis-

---

1   The brown color is the complexion of the people who presently inhabit the Near Eastern region, the Biblical and geographical location of the Garden of Eden (Gen. 2:7–15),the lost home of Adam & Eve.

perse to other areas. There was a great human movement and migration of companies and families from the Near East to other parts of the world (Gen. 11:7–9). Families and companies with identical skin color and with hearing and speaking skills for a "tongue", naturally, moved out in search of geographical location for the survival and preservation of the culture and independence of the group (Gen. 10:6, 20). How and when the various racial groups settled in their respective geographical zones and continents is mere conjecture and beyond the scope of this work.

The word of God, however, informs us that God "determined the times set for them and the exact places where they should live" (Acts 17:26; cf. Deut. 32:8; Dan. 4:35). The territorial allocation for the dispersed groups is not meant to isolate one group from the other. The Apostle Paul suggests that the reason for that allotment is to offer the groups the opportunity to seek the Lord (Acts 17:27). Each color group is to seek the Lord from its respective place of habitation. God's presence is to be felt and acknowledged anywhere and everywhere around the corners of the earth, and where there is human life. Each color group is to "reach out" to find God, around whom the entire color groups meet to praise, and in whom the color differences are dissolved.

In one of his visions of the throne of God, John the revealer describes what he saw in the following words: "After these things I looked, and behold, a great multitude which no one could number, of all nations, tribes, peoples, and tongues, standing before the throne, and before the Lamb, clothed with white robes, with palm branches in their hands, and crying with a loud voice, saying, 'salvation belongs to our God who sits on the throne, and to the Lamb'" (Rev. 7:9–10, NKJV).

The apostle John saw great multitudes of men and women of all the nations of the world. Redeemed from every tribal, language, and racial groups—the Caucasoid, the Mongoloid, the Negroid, etc.—stood before the holy God on His throne and before the Lamb, Jesus Christ. Remember, dear reader that the unholy and the sinful cannot stand before the holy God, but John saw the black complexioned, the light, and the brown-yellow colored saints, all proud and equal before God (Rev. 7: 9–17; 14:1–5).

Common Features of all Creation

For one thing, both the theory of African ancestors of the human race and the biblical accounts of creation give credence to the fact that all skin colors come from the same source. There is nothing intrinsically evil with any of the skin colors, and none is either inferior or superior to the other, because all the skin colors are organically linked or bonded. The three coloring matters, which affect or determine human skin color—melanin, melanoid, and carotene—are all found in the black-colored African, as well as in the light-colored European, and in the brown-yellow-colored Chinese and North American Indian. The variety in the human skin color results from distinctive amount or quantity of the pigment dominant in each group of the human race (see Harold Cummins, "Skin Color", *Collier's Encyclopedia*, Vol. 21, New York: Collier's, 1997, 63. Cf. Arkady Leokum, *the Big Book of Tell Me Why*, New York: Purlieu Press, 1989, 117–118)

There is only one kind of human flesh (1 Cor. 15:39), but generated in many colors.

All creation in heaven and on earth, both living and non-living, animals, and plants, are made in different shapes and colors. In spite of their color variations, the beast and the birds, for example, instinctively, live in harmony, and project with their varied skin colors a common beauty, and a world of attraction for the admiration of the human race.

Similarly, the plant world with their differences in shape and color displays harmony, beauty, and healing for other creation.

Humanity is a part and, in fact, the crowning act of God's creation. Humanity, therefore, would share with the common features of all the other creatures. The variation in human skin color should be seen as a purposeful and distinctive design for mankind as an integral part of God's creation.

Skin Color and the Climate

Many scientists and, particularly, the evolutionists, explain the differences in human skin color as structural adaptations to different climatic conditions on earth. They believe, for example that the black skin is suited for a hot climate, and that the melanin, a substance responsible for dark skin, is designed to protect the skin from the harsh or excessive heat of the sun. On the other hand light skin color has the absorbing and regulating property for a cold weather. It is further believed that the genetic composition of the various groups of the human race naturally changes to meet up with changes in the weather or climate. This belief credits the climate as the determinant factor for the variation in human skin color. This belief is confirmed by the theory of natural selection; a contention that only the organism best fitted for or genetically adapted to a specific environment can survive. The organism's traits are naturally passed on to its offspring.

If skin color is associated with the climate, do we, therefore, expect in the next millions of years some dramatic evolutionary change of the skin color of the black Africans who now live in the temperate zone, and vice versa of the light colored who live in the tropical regions of the earth? The lack of evidence of a change in the skin color of, for example, a fifteenth-century immigrant and his/her twenty-first century offspring in spite of change in climate and geographical location, would question the association of skin color with the climate. Besides, the belief that all three skin-coloring substances are present in every human being should lead to a more sober reflection of the purpose for the various human skin colors. Obviously, the human skin color is more than a structural adaptation to the climate.

The Significance of Human Skin Colors

In the following words, "Let us make man in our image, according to our likeness" (Gen. 1:26, NKJV), we read the divine declaration that man came into being not by happenstance, but by God's plan and design. God was willing to share his existence with man. He liberally endowed man with elements of personality similar to his.

God is a perfect Being (Matt. 5:48). Everything about him and from him is perfect. His thoughts and gifts for man in particular, and his other creation generally, are good and perfect. The Apostle James says, "Every good gift and every perfect gift is from above and cometh down from the father of lights, with whom is no variables, neither shadow of turning" (James 1:17, KJV). All that man is in form or structure and color is God's best, and reflects his wisest choice for man, the very masterpiece of his creation.

Every inventor or manufacturer has a trademark for his product. The trademark shows the origin and ownership of a product, and gives the manufacturer or merchant an exclusive right to his product. For the conservative Christian, man is an indisputable product of the hand of God. Does God have a trademark for his product? Of course He does. The skin color is an inextricable part of the human body, and can be seen as God's trademark of his creation in humankind.

The skin color of every racial group is an indelible mark of identity, and colorful expression to the cultural adaptations and practices of the group. The human skin color is designed to awaken in every man a personal and meditational reflection of the mystery in his creation and being. The human skin color leads us to believe in and look at the self as a unique creation, and to appreciate the beauty in variety. The varied skin colors are meant to arouse in us an awareness and acknowledgement of the intelligence and artistic work of the divine Sculptor or potter, and painter. The human skin color is, above all, a structural adaptation to the worship and service of God. The colors are put in place to meet his divine purpose. The Apostle Paul counsels, "Present your bodies as a living sacrifice, holy and pleasing to God. This is your spiritual act of worship" (Rom.12: 1).

It is an act of worship to glorify God in our body. To glorify God in our body includes reflecting the holiness and unchanging personality of God. To reflect, through appreciation and maintenance of the natural texture of the skin, what God believes in and expects from his creation. God believes that his creation is distinct and good. Therefore, He requires from man a reciprocal mental attitude of belief and confidence in him/herself. Every one should see himself or herself as a complete and perfect piece of God's handiwork that needs no makeup or adjustment.

Besides, Paul's counsel was a re-echo of God's word in the book of Leviticus 22:20–24. God requires a living sacrifice, non-defective and physically perfect. The act of presenting a sacrificial animal with a physical abnormality displeases God. Whereas, sacrifice is an act of giving up what one may consider indispensable and which under normal circumstances could not be given up. Therefore, the Christian should be willing to give up that cherished physical and outward display, because in worship God wants to meet with the simple and natural, not the superficial man.

Human skin color is an acid test today, a test of acceptance and belief that God's work can neither be modified nor improved upon. It is also a stumbling block for those who act in denial of a universal brotherhood and sisterhood of all the color groups of the human race

A concept about the place and significance of skin color is developed from the prayer of three young men at a musical concert. Three men, each representing a color group were invited for a musical program. At the end of their presentation, they held hands together, bowed and prayed, "Thank you God for making me what I am, and for whom we are by the talents given to each one, for your honor and glory, Amen." The prayer appreciates the uniqueness of each person, and expresses a common Creator for the three. It also recognizes that whatever one is and has is a gift which should be used for the glory of the Creator God.

Every one has a measure of the skin coloring substances found in others. Thus, while we are physically unique by the visible color of our skin, the internal bond of the coloring substances relates us all. According to this belief what a person is by color has meaning and value only in relation to persons of other color group. Our perfect God could not have given any man an imperfect colored skin without running the risk of being an imperfect and partial God. God's choice for man cannot be questioned. It is the best for man. The prophet Isaiah quotes, "For my thoughts are not your thoughts, neither are your ways my ways, declares the Lord. As the heavens are higher than the earth so are my ways higher than your ways, and my thoughts than your thoughts" (Isa. 55:8, 9). Our sovereign God gives and does whatever pleases Him (Ps. 135:6).

The all-knowing and all-powerful God chose for Himself the form and color of man. Man had no choice over his position as a creature. However, man exercises his power of choice over that which pertains to or affects his relationship with God, and with his fellow creatures. For example, Mr. Timberwolve could choose to be a Christian, but could not choose his parents. Neither could he choose his language, tribal or racial group, nor the color of his skin. God, the Creator, made this choice for Timberwolve, the creature. Timberwolve can choose or decide at any moment not to be a Christian. But he cannot choose or decide not to be a brown-yellow colored man, because he has even deep in his bone marrow, all that it takes to be an American Indian.

What does it take to be either black or a light-colored person?

For a traditional African, it may take merely a wish for a desired complexion. For instance, a traditional African couple that was married for twelve years had their fourth child, a baby girl with fairer skin color. The man accused his wife of infidelity and rejected the girl as his because she resembled none of the man's family members.

In the absence of a DNA test, the man consulted with the village Native Doctor/Seer. The Seer claimed that the baby was the man's dead aunt who has been re-incarnated. The man's aunt was fair in complexion, and had died sixty years earlier before the birth of the girl. But shortly before her death she expressed a wish to retain her complexion in her next world. Perhaps the workings of heredity would unscramble the puzzle. However the issue before us is not a question of hereditary but a question of the source of skin colors.

Let us assume there is a medical break-through for extracting and replacing dominant or paired recessive gene from one skin color to a different skin color. Can medical science produce light skin out of brown-yellow colored man, and vice versa, as a result of the infusion of or replacement with dominant gene or sufficient quantity of pigment for the desired skin color? There is more to skin color than its genetic makeup or carriers.

Does it take a certain type of blood to be what one is in color? Of course not, because blood donated, for example, by Timberwolve, an American Indian, to Mr. Bia, a black African, cannot have any changing effects on Bia's skin pigment. Mr. Bia cannot cease to be a black African on account of the blood donated from the American Indian. It does not take hair color, or geographical location to be what you are in color. It neither takes cloning nor skin grafting to be what and how you are in color. The indisputable truth of the matter is that it takes God's choice and creation to be what we are in physical form and color. Every man and woman should see him/herself as divinely clothed with a second-to-none or superior-to-none skin color for a life of honor and dignity to his/her human race in general, and color group in particular.

Another fact to note about our human body is that death and resurrection cannot alter the skin color. The Apostle Paul hinted at this in his treatise on the resurrection. In his answer to an objection against the resurrection of the dead, Paul made this analogy, "What you sow is not made alive unless it dies. What you sow, you do not sow that body that shall be, but mere grain—perhaps wheat or some other grain. God gives it a body as He pleases, and to each seed its own body" (1 Cor. 15:36–38, NKJV).

A farmer who sows, for example, a yellow corn would expect to harvest a fresh yellow corn. The fresh corn may look differently from the old one in its shape or form. But the identity of the planted seed is retained and preserved in the fresh seed. Unless there is cross-pollination with different species, the corn would retain its yellowish color. The corn will always be corn with a distinct body of its own given to it by God as it pleased Him. Paul's analogy illustrates the fact that there is an organic link between the dead and the resurrected body. The organic link is not lost in death

It is not mere speculation to say that a man's skin color will be an identifying mark or feature by which the man will be known and recognized in a recreated and restored Eden. Paul might have alluded to this fact when he wrote, "For now we see through a glass darkly, but then, face to face, now I know in part, but then shall I know even as also I am known" (1 Cor. 13:12, KJV).

Ede was born a black man. He is subject to death as a black man. He will be raised from the grave on the resurrection morning with a black complexion. If he accepts by faith the sacrifice of Jesus Christ, his Redeemer, and lives a life of obedience to His will, he will be a black man saved by grace. His color identity now will neither be lost in death nor at the resurrection. But wait a moment; didn't the word of God indicate that the redeemed would be changed at the second coming of Jesus Christ? "Behold, I tell you a mystery. We shall not all sleep, but we shall be changed, in a moment, in the twinkling of an eye, at the last trump. For the trumpet will sound, and the dead will be raised incorruptible, and we shall be changed" (1 Cor. 15: 51–53, NKJV). Surely, the redeemed will be changed. However, what would be changed is not the color of the skin. Every human body, presently, is subject to decay and rottenness. On the resurrection day, the righteous dead will rise with the original skin color they had before death. The skin color of the redeemed will be indestructible in the sense that it is not something attached to the skin or body, which can be rubbed off or skinned out. It is the texture of the skin or body. The redeemed will not be given a skin color entirely different from the one they had at birth. The change refers to the fact that both the righteous living and their resurrected counterparts will no longer be subject to death and decay. We now have mortal bodies, but at the second coming of Jesus the mortal will be changed to glorified and immortal body. And every redeemed man and woman, of whatever complexion, will live in eternity before the eternal presence of God.

There is yet another fact to consider in reference to the state of our skin color. The Apostle Paul penned the following, "Therefore, just as sin entered the world through one man, and death through sin, and in this way death came to all men, because all sinned" (Rom. 5:12). All are born in sin, and all are under the bondage of sin. All stand before God condemned. All flesh is subject to death. But Jesus on behalf of the entire human race paid the penalty for sin. It is the shed blood on the cross, not the skin color that covers the sin-infested flesh (Rom. 5:6–9). The redeeming love and death of Jesus is all-inclusive. It includes the Caucasoid, the Mongoloid, the Negroid, etc., for Jesus sees in every man something worth dying for. His all-inclusive death implies his intense desire for the eternal continuity of the human race with its varied skin color.

In one of his visions of the metropolis of the New World, John writes: "And the *nations* of those who are saved shall walk in its light, and the kings of the earth bring their glory and honor in it...and they shall bring the glory and honor of the *nations* into it...In the middle of its streets and on the other side of the river, was the tree of life which bore twelve fruits, each tree yielding its fruit every month. The leaves of the tree were for the healing of the *nations* (Rev. 21:24, 26; 22:2, NKJV). John did not mince words when he affirmed that the saved of all nations, the representatives of all human skin colors, tongues and trives, shall walk in the fadeless light of the metropolis of the New World. The health-sustaining leaves and fruits of the tree of life are within the reach of all. The saved, irrespective of his/her skin color, is given the right to live and move freely. Every one of the redeemed of all colors and nations is a king with and subject only to God.

In retrospect, God created mankind with varied colors He is proud with His creation.

Every human skin color is God's choice and identity for, and stamp of ownership on his creation. The mark or stamp is for life and eternity beyond the grave. The varied colors reflect order and organization in creation, rather than confusion and division among his creatures. The various human skin colors are designed to humble us and arouse that sense and feeling of the awesomeness of God. Besides, the ingenuity shown in the formation of the clay/dust into living beings with colored skin is incomprehensible. It reveals the supreme Mind and master designer.

We are vessels fashioned unto honor. God places a price tag on every vessel. That price tag is, irrespective of color, the blood of Jesus Christ.

Meeting some Beliefs about Black Skin

The Bible gives an account of a universal flood long ago. There were then no coast guards, no firefighters, and no helicopters to help save millions of lives that were drowned in that flood (Gen. 7:11, 12, 23, 24). But there was only one family of eight that survived through the flood. This family was comprised of a father, Noah with his wife and three children. Each of the children had a wife. Noah's sons were Shem, Ham, and Japhet. Ham is believed to be the progenitor of the black-colored group of the human race. The sons of Ham include Cush (Ethiopia), Mizraim (Egypt), Put (Libya), and Canaan (Gen. 10:6).

An incident in the life of Noah, and the reaction of his son, Ham to that incident changed or affected the course of history. The Bible reports the incident in the following words, "And Noah began to be a farmer, and he planted a vineyard. Then he drank of the wine and was drunk, and became uncovered in his tent. Ham, the father of Canaan, saw the nakedness of his father, and told his brothers outside. But Shem and Japhet took a garment, laid it on their shoulders, and went backward and covered the nakedness of their father. Their faces were turned away, and they did not see their father's nakedness" (Gen. 9: 20–30, NKJV)

Ham probably made fun of his father's nakedness before his brothers. That was considered a dishonor to a father. When Noah awoke from his sleep and found out what his youngest son had done to him, he said, "Cursed be Canaan. The lowest of slaves would he be to his brothers" (Gen. 9:24, 25). It is not within the scope of this book to discuss why Canaan, instead of Ham, the culprit, was cursed. But the saying, "The fathers have eaten sour grapes, and the children's teeth are set on edge" (Ezek. 18:2; Jer. 31: 29, 30, NKJV), seems to be true of Ham with his son, Canaan. Ham dishonored his father, Noah. But Noah pronounced a curse upon Canaan his grandson.

Some see this curse as extended to and/or inherited by the black people, particularly the black Africans. The slave trade is seen as a fulfillment of that curse, and reinforcement to the belief that the black-colored group of the human race is a cursed and inferior group. Many, by words and action, associate black skin with slavery. Some black persons have been conditioned to think and believe that their skin color is a mark of slavery and inferiority. Hence, some modern men and women of African descent, in their desire to look like others with skin color different from theirs, or in the name of fashion, resort to bleaching creams, and/or skin lighteners. They also resort to changing their hair color.

Looking at the whole issue of slavery of the black Africans, we see openly displayed man's engagements in history. The ancient African kings and traditional elders that engaged in inter and intra-tribal wars for slaves received no mandate of Heaven for their ignominious activities. Their cooperation with the Arabs and European slave dealers, undoubtedly, a factor that encouraged slave trade was a choice they made with no coercion. In fact without their full cooperation and active support there would have been blank pages in history for a slave trade that never was.

Secondly, the black African who was physically and emotionally separated from his native land had many disadvantages in a foreign land. His helplessness and disadvantages were effectively manipulated by his master in order to control his will for a perpetual servitude. The slave master built him a Church not to save but enslave his soul. A systematic Bible teaching, leading to a theology of submission was developed. The pulpit was regularly used as a platform for indoctrination, preaching, and teaching master-superiority. The slaves were daily reminded of Christian virtues of obedience and loyalty to human authority.

Further, black skin was made an object of caricature and derogation in the media. There was, indeed, a relentless verbal, physical and psychological thrust to de-humanize the black African, and condition him into believing that slavery was the best and only option for him. For time slavery became an indispensable part of social structure for meeting the people's need for recognition and power. As a part of social structure of the day, and with many centuries of its practice slavery was ingrained in the economic culture of the people. To give up slavery would amount to economic suicide for many slave masters.

In fact the civil war that rocked the very existence of the United States of America was an aftermath of intransigent stance for slavery in the southern states of the country.

The black African slavery is one of the many in recorded history. The Bible and secular history testify to the fact that man's enslavement to and by his fellow man, irrespective of skin color, is an age-long practice. Kings and nobles of ancient empires of the world, for example, have had many of their fellow citizens subjected to slavery.

In view of this fact of history, one can confidently contend that slave trade with its dehumanizing abuses and derogatory implications to the black Africans was not a result of any curse on the black people. The enslavement was prompted by an economic survival and exploitative ambitions of the colonists. The Africans had proved in their native lands to be hardworking and strongly built to survive through harsh conditions.

Thus, when the need for a strong and stable work force arose in the Americas, the Africans were sought for and taken to replace the Native Americans.

The enslaved Africans were neither street boys and girls nor mean men and women. They were established and responsible citizens who needed nothing but security, peace and quietude in their native land. Among them were geniuses, intelligent and creative. These Africans lost all but their minds and skills when they left the shores of Africa in chains.

Their skills, intelligence, and creativity enriched and sustained in no small measure the social and spiritual life of the Americas.

The slave masters' high-handedness, social isolation and deprivations of basic human rights had their toll on the Africans, adversely distorting their perception of themselves and the society. The ensuing circumstantial shortcomings and weaknesses of the slaves were interpreted by the society as inherent of a people with black skin.

As a matter of fact no other racial group could fare differently and better with stigma of slavery and sub-human conditions as the black Africans. In fact if roles and social status of the European slave masters and their African slaves are swapped or reversed, the outcome is predictable. Mankind needs right and favorable conditions and opportunities to be and to develop fully. If and when this need is denied, no one, whatever skin color or language group can scale beyond the level of slavery without a sustained fight.

Reflection on the factors that prompted slavery yields nothing to suggest a curse or a divine approval. Therefore, the "curse" mentality and belief of some people is not only a rationalization for arrogance and justification for slavery but unsound exegetical application of the curse of Noah's grandson (see Gen. 9:24–29). A belief that God created but did not destine and set up any racial group to be cursed leads to a conviction that the black-colored group of the human race is not under an inherited curse. A close examination of all the curses mentioned in the Bible leads to the conclusion that 1) a curse may either be an immediate response to or a predictive result of a sinful act, and disobedience to God's directive; 2) every curse is conditional, and personal because once cursed is not forever cursed; and 3) a curse may be turned into a blessing by repentance and obedience. It is one's moral character, and not one's physical appearance or complexion that would lead to either a curse or a blessing; 4) God does not punish a guiltless son for the sins of his father (Ezek. 18:20). However, every flesh, be it black or light or brown-yellow is under the curse of sin.

"For as many as are of the works of the law are under the curse of sin; for it is written, 'Cursed is every one who does not continue in all things which are written in the book of the law, to do them'" (Gal. 3:10, NKJV, cf. Deut. 11:26; 27:15–26; Lev. 26:1–14; Prov.3:33).

In contrast, "Blessed are those who do his commandments that they may have the right to the tree of life, and may enter through the gates into the city" (Rev. 22:14). There is a curse, irrespective of skin color, upon one who breaks the law of God.

Many, as a symbol of evil or sin, generally see the black color. Satan is presented and represented always as black colored. If Lucifer is a dark-complexioned being, then there should be no reason to dispute the belief that black skin originated with God. The word of God presents Lucifer in his unfallen state as a perfect and beautiful created being (Ezek. 28:11–15). Lucifer could have been a light-colored being in heaven before his rebellion. He could not have evolved later into a black-colored being after his rebellion. He would either be dark colored or light colored before and after his rebellion and fall.

What is the skin color of the angelic host in heaven? The Bible intimates that every child of God has a guardian angel (Heb. 1:14). Naturally, as a black person, I would expect my guardian angel to appear, and identify with me, as a black ministering Spirit. However, in heaven and in earth made new, the joy of salvation will turn or overshadow every skin color into insignificance.

The identification of black skin with evil, and the overt and covert rejection of the black skin, has no factual and scriptural basis. The black men and women who were used by God for His cause both in the Old and New Testament times call to question the erroneous beliefs, and negative attitude towards black complexion.

The Black Men and Women of the Bible

One of the inspired books of the Bible, "The Song of Solomon", is devoted entirely to discussing a dramatic love story of King Solomon and his black Shulamite bride. The Shulamite damsel describes herself as "black", but lovely" (Song of Sol. 1:5, 6). King Solomon adds, "O thou fairest among women; behold thou art fair, my love; behold thou art fair; thou hast doves' eyes" (Song of Sol. 1:8, 15, KJV). The swarthy complexion of the Shulamite girl is further confirmed and illustrated by the use of such metaphors as "tents of Kedar" (Song of Sol. 1:5); "pillars of smoke" (Song of Sol. 3:6); and "black hair as a flock of goats" (Song of Sol. 4:1; 6:5).

The love story is seen as either figurative of God's love for the people of ancient Israel, or an allegory of Christ's love for His bride, the Christian Church. Whatever is the right or generally accepted interpretation to the story, there is one outstanding fact in the book.

The culturally biased biblical expositors and interpreters may ignore the fact because it condemns negative thinking and discontent for black complexion. The Shulamite girl is a symbol of either God's covenant people of ancient Israel or Christ's bride, the Christian Church. The figure of a black woman for God's people should awaken our dull and slumbering mind to comprehend God's inclusiveness in His salvation economy. That inclusiveness is further demonstrated by God's use of some black men and women for special duties on behalf of God's people in the Old and New Testament era.

The Holy Spirit preserved for our reference the names of those black men and women who were actively involved in the cause of God for the ancient Israel and for the Christian Church today. The first in the list is Jethro, the Priest of Midian. Jethro was black, and God-fearing man. The success of Moses as a leader and administrator should be credited in part to the wise and timely advice of his father in-law. At a critical moment of his son in-law's career Jethro became a management consultant, and advisor to Moses.

It was from Jethro that Moses learnt and put to use some management and administrative principles for the arduous task of leading the horde of indiscipline and rebellious wanderers (Exod. 3:1; 18:1, 17–26). Jethro's principles of management are still relevant today. In every age and society leaders and administrators have adopted, and adapted to those principles with optimum success.

The next black person in the list was Zipporah, the wife of Moses, and Jethro's daughter (Exod. 2:21; 18:2). The Bible presents her as an Ethiopian (Num. 12:1, KJV). As the daughter of God-fearing priest, Zipporah evidently exercised a positive influence upon Moses. Zipporah proved to be a courageous and reliable companion and helper in time of crisis. Her courage in the face of a life-threatening confrontation was dramatic: "And the Lord said to Moses, when you go back to Egypt, see that you do all those wonder before Pharaoh which I have put in your mind... and it came to pass on the way, at the encampment, that the Lord met him (Moses) and sought to kill him. Zipporah took a sharp stone and cut off the foreskin of her son and cast it at Moses' feet, and said, 'Surely you are a husband of blood to me'" (Exod. 4:21, 24, 25). Moses had either forgotten or neglected to heed to the injunction of God to circumcise his male children. The negligence of the injunction incurred God's wrath. Zipporah's swift intervention and courage to circumcise their son with an improvised object or instruments saved the day for her husband. Zipporah removed an object of offense to God. Thus, the life of Moses was spared for the cause of God among his chosen people of Israel.

Another person on the line of some black men and women, who were actively involved in God's salvation economy, was also a woman. Her name was Jael, the wife of Heber, a descendant of Jethro. Jael bravely helped to put an end to the reign of terror perpetuated by Sisera, the captain of Jabin, a Canaanite king who oppressed Israel (Judg. 4:11, 17, 21). The Prophetess, and female Judge, Deborah, says of Jael, "Blessed above women shall Jael, the wife of Heber, the Kenite be...blessed shall she be above women in the tent...She put her hand to the nail, and her right hand to the workmen's hammer; and with the hammer she smote Sisera...(Judg. 5:24, 26, KJV). In Jael, a remarkable housewife, God found a willing heart and hand who without formal solicitation from any one, moved fearlessly and swiftly to put an end to the human instrument of oppression. Jael's action cut short the tide of the battle for the victory and liberation of God's covenant people.

In the New Testament, the contributions of Simon, the Cyrene, are not overlooked.

The Holy Spirit preserved for generations of men the record of Simon's, ministry. When Jesus had not enough strength to carry the cross, He found in Simon an empathizer who endured shame to carry the Savior's cross. By carrying that cross, Simon publicly identified himself with the person and cause of Jesus Christ.

What do we make out of this reference to these black men and women of the Bible times? In God's salvation economy the black colored men and women are called and used for important, and sometimes dangerous tasks. God in many ways has demonstrated His love for and acceptance of man irrespective of color.

To recapitulate the basic argument of the chapter, the following points are underscored:

- The human skin color is neither determined through the evolution process nor the result of exposure to the climate or weather but by the creation of God.

- The skin colors are to be traced back to one source. To those who accept the theory of African origin of human life, the one source is the "African Eve". And for those who accept the biblical account of creation, all skin colors should be traced back to Adam and Eve, the progenitors of the human race.

- Every skin color is a blend of melanin, melanoid and carotene. These three coloring substances disproportionately blend to give mankind its various complexions. The differences in color, shape, and form or structure are special features which all creatures—human, beasts, plants, etc.—have in common. These features have been determined by a force or power outside the man, or the beast, and the plant. For the Bible-believing Christian, that power is God. Besides, it has been observed that no two persons, except identical twins, look exactly alike. Thus, difference in structure and complexion from one racial group to another is nature's design. We have no choice but to appreciate the varied human complexions.

- No one should be preoccupied with color of the skin but with the place and contribution of one's complexion in the creation and salvation economy of God.

The various points made about human complexion suggest that any act of "improving" the complexion by the use of lighteners or other beauty preparations cannot be commended by God. The act reveals low self-esteem, and a misuse of an opportunity to acknowledge the magnanimous gift of God. Besides, any hateful act influenced by ethnocentric biases or otherwise contradicts a belief in a Creator God in whose image and likeness mankind was made.

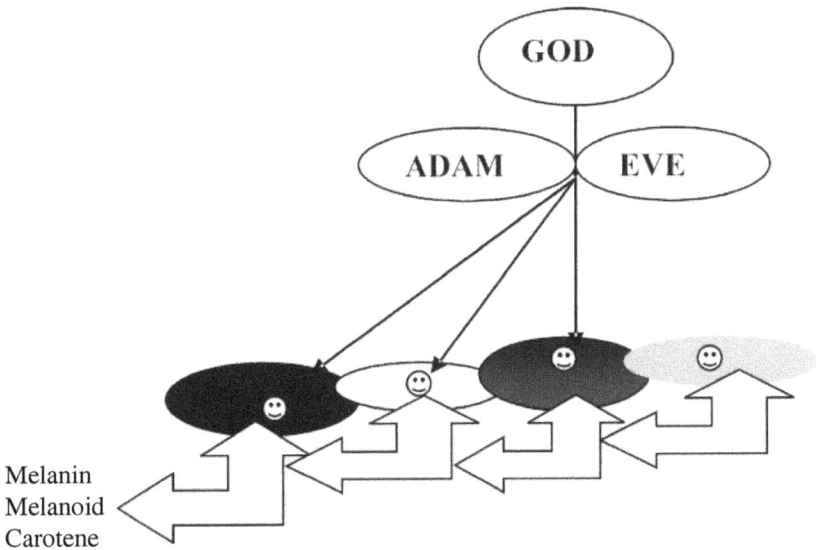

Melanin
Melanoid
Carotene

The source and inter-relatedness of all skin colors

My Skin

Like an elegant dress of a million dollar.
Tailored and worn from a mother's womb
Seamless but colored to match
Its texture a feel of ingenuity
Its design a masterpiece of its designer
An all-season outfit mine to wear
Till time renders it a treasured memorabilia
To mend or soil I must not. For its designer will visit
the dog that values no sacred dress.

CHAPTER 3

REACTIONS TO HUMAN SKIN COLOR

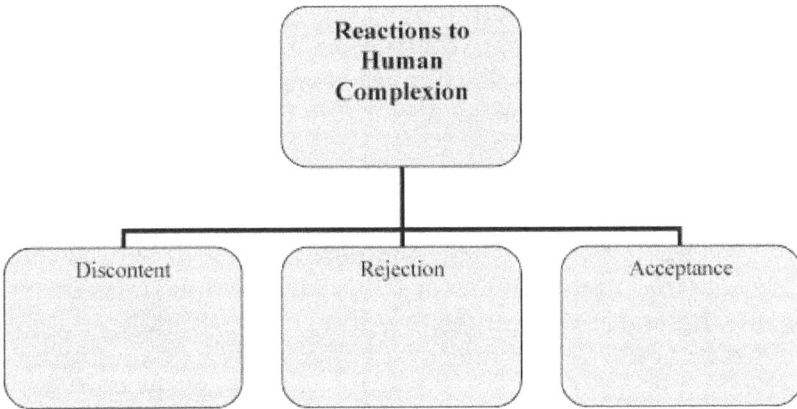

```
                    ┌─────────────────┐
                    │  Reactions to   │
                    │     Human       │
                    │   Complexion    │
                    └────────┬────────┘
          ┌──────────────────┼──────────────────┐
  ┌───────────────┐  ┌───────────────┐  ┌───────────────┐
  │   Discontent  │  │   Rejection   │  │   Acceptance  │
  └───────────────┘  └───────────────┘  └───────────────┘
```

Motivations

1. Ethnic biases and/or prejudice
2. Social pressure
3. Desire for acceptance and/or admiration
4. Lust
5. Love

Social Approach to Human Complexion

1. Makeup/cosmetics
2. surgery
3. hate/hostility
4. love/acceptance

An Eyewitness account:

Ede was born and raised in a rural African tribal village with a population of less than ten thousand families. The population was mainly made up of peasant farmers. The only world Ede knew, as a little boy was his tribal village. For him

29

everything began and ended in his village. He saw and lived with no other group, but his own ethnic and racial group. No one was different from his mom and dad. Ede was socially, emotionally and mentally attached to and tucked into his cultural block. However, at five, Ede's world and horizon began to expand beyond the common sites and people he used to visit and play with. Other villages and towns came into his view, but the people from the surrounding villages and towns looked no different either. At the age of seven, he developed doubts about what he used to know and believe as a homogeneous world. Ede was taught the "white" man's language, but he had never seen or met any "white" man. He longed for the day when he would see and speak with the white man.

Not long after his eighth birthday, a religious camp meeting was held near his village. And for the first time in his life Ede saw and met with Pastor Clifford, a "white" missionary from England. Ede's inquisitive and curious mind could not be held back when he and other boys shyly and timidly approached Pastor Clifford. When Pastor Clifford stretched out his hand for a handshake, Ede nervously but joyfully held and rubbed the white man's hairy hand. Ede sat close as possible to Pastor Clifford and watched every movement he made. He saw the white man smile, talk, and sing. The white man's song, "Jesus loves the little children. All the children of the world, red and yellow, black and white, are precious in his sight", made a deep impression and raised some questions in his mind about skin colors. By the end of the day, Ede had reached a conclusion. Pastor Clifford, the white man, was as human as his dad. The only visible difference was the color of his skin. In his childlike innocence and curiosity, Ede approached and asked Pastor Clifford, "Why is your skin color different from every other person here in the camp?" "God made me so," Pastor Clifford replied. "And me too?" Ede retorted. "Yes, God made us all," Clifford responded.

Many years later Ede visited the Scandinavian country of Sweden for a summer as a student. He had the privilege to visit and make calls to many Swedish homes in the countryside, and summer homes. One of those calls turned out to be an unpleasant experience. In his moment of reflection of the day's work and activities, that experience brought him an embarrassing memory of human reactionary behavior to an unfamiliar object.

On approaching one home in the countryside of Skruv, a small railroad town, Ede saw a little boy by a tractor. A few yards away from the tractor was the little boy's mother. When the little boy, named Gunnar, saw Ede he screamed, jumped out of the tractor and ran towards his mother. Gunnar tucked in his head under the arms of his mother, to keep his eyes away from the strange man. When he looked again and saw Ede walking towards them, he struggled to release himself from his mother to a more secure and hidden place in the house. It took a mother's calm posture and persuasion to calm the physically shaken boy. "The boy has not seen a black person before," the mother explained.

"He just could not stand the sight of a strange looking figure at this hour of the day," she added. The little Gunnar looked at Ede from head to toes with suspicion and uneasiness. After a short sales talk with the little boy's mother, a set of the children's bedtime stories was bought for the little Gunnar. The gift of a book from Ede, a black man, eased Gunnar's tension, and changed the atmosphere of suspicion to tolerance. Amused by the boy's reaction to his skin color, Ede became conscious of his color, and cautious in every home he visited.

Barely three weeks later, Ede had an experience dissimilar to his encounter with Gunnar. Ede came to a home and pressed the doorbell. The door was immediately swung open. As the door opened, Ede saw a woman in her late seventies, standing before him. After a brief introduction of himself in a mumbled and memorized Swedish words [*Svenska*],

Ede was invited in and offered a cold drink. A brief sales talk did not yield any sale.

However, the woman engaged Ede in conversation. Ede discovered that the woman was a widow. In the previous years she had offered accommodation to several African students, in spite of their skin color. She treated them kindly. A track of mails confirmed unbroken communications between Elsa Bergman, the Swedish angel, and the African students.

Ede's childhood curiosity over a white missionary's skin color, and his bittersweet experience as an African student were relived many years later. After his college education, Ede took up a temporary appointment as a substitute teacher. During his first assignment as a substitute for a bilingual class teacher, he met with a group of seven-year old children. In their free time some of the children went behind Ede to touch his black hair. When he objected, one of the kids asked, "Maestro [teacher], where are you from?"

Ede replied, "From heaven." The kids responded in unison, "No, you are from Africa, or the Island, or...

"Ede's experience from childhood to his adulthood is presented to illustrate some reactions to human skin colors. From the case before us we see three major reactions: 1) childhood curiosity that led Ede and some of his seven-year-old students touch to feel the skin and hair of someone of a different skin and hair color; 2) Gunnar's childish and temporary aversion for a person of color; and 3) the widow's acceptance and accommodation of persons from a different color group.

Factors influencing Reactions:

The reactions mentioned above, with the exception of the childlike curiosity to touch and feel the skin and hair of someone, have one common underlying factor. This common factor is that they are learned behaviors. They are not genetically determined or inherited. In the case of the little boy, Gunnar, it was fear of an unfamiliar object. Probably, that fear was learned from either or both of his parents. Our attitude towards life is generally learned from the environment. The home lays the groundwork for tolerance and accommodation or rejection and hostility to the colored persons. Childish aversion for a colored person, for example, may be reinforced, strengthened or weakened as years go by

The home climate or environment and other factors such as peer groups and one's choice play a part in influencing attitude towards people or things. The one reaction or attitude that needs further evaluation is the aversion for a colored person.

An aversion for colored people is displayed in many ways, some subtle and some openly. Some of the ways include violent physical acts, such as homicide and arson.

Another subtle way is a denial of employment and promotion of qualified candidates on the basis of their skin color and ethnic background. These aversive acts that defy comprehension and imagination are, without doubt, motivated by hatred. They are by their nature and intent, "hate crime.

Hate crimes include prejudging someone by the color of his/her skin. It is an open secret that many have been shot and dragged to death on first sight for no apparent reason other than their skin color and/or accent. There are professed Christians that are biased by the complexion and accent of their fellows. These professed Christians may conceal their anger and hate with a lively handshake and a broad smile on meeting their victims. They are quick to criticize and condemn, and would see nothing good from the hated color and language group. Common human errors of the hated ones are seen as unpardonable. And treated with all severity the hated persons or color and language groups do not deserve.

Hate crimes may result from an unmet or unfulfilled psychological need for attention and recognition. The perpetrators of hate crimes may feel good and proud about their actions, because the attention they do not normally get is eventually received from the society for their mischievous and diabolical acts. Hate crimes may be a result of pride based on false or real assumptions of superiority. An assumed superiority that is based, for example, on the historical events of slavery may not be easily outgrown in a capitalist economy and society. The proud and ill informed that has been exposed to constantly hearing and using cultural or racial slur and epithets perceives and treats the colored as inferior. He is self-conceited in what he perceives as his domain of authority over the persons. On the other hand, a feeling of inferiority may not be ruled out as a factor that encourages hostility. One who feels inadequate and intimidated may do one of several things. He may hide his feelings by engaging in a heinous act within or without his racial or language group, an act that he believes would project him as a hero among his people. He may tend to withdraw from people and only to be identified with a heinous act against the persons he perceives as the source of his inadequacy.

Language-phobia Factor:

Hate crime is "color" based as well as "language" motivated. Language and cultural differences have often led to political rivalries, suspicion and distrust among ethnic groups, particularly, in the developing nations of the world. Intra-racial and ethnic conflicts in most cases are very bloody. Lives and materials are wasted. Social developments are crippled, and progress at all levels of human endeavors is hampered.

Evidently, professed Christians and adherents of other religions of the world support and carry out these hostilities. Some give assent to or connive at evil against their fellow believers who are culturally and linguistically different. Unfortunately, too, Churches, Mosque, and temples are turned into slaughtering houses for the victims of ethnic biases and hatred. Likewise ethnocentric feeling has often led to contempt and discrimination of a language group. This is a serious disregard of a historical fact in the Scriptures. The Bible writer reports: "Now the whole world had one language and a common speech. As men moved eastward, they found a plain in Shinar and settled there....Then they said, 'come let us build ourselves a city, with a tower that reaches to the heavens, so that we may make a name for ourselves and not be scattered over the face of the whole earth' The Lord said if as one people speaking the same language they have begun to do this, then nothing they plan to do will be impossible for them. Come, let us go down and confuse their language so they will not understand each other" (Genesis 11:1, 2, 4, 6, 7). Either this Scriptural text is true or the entire Bible is make-believe of human encounter in history with God. I certainly believe God's written word to be true and accurate.

The postdiluvian world with one common language conspired to build a self-contained empire on a foundation of godlessness. It was a sort of mob confrontation with and resistance to God's authority. However, God has a thousand ways of getting his plans through in spite of man's opposition. God introduced numerous languages and gave men differing utterances. The one common language was made obsolete. The tower builders could no longer understand each other. The mass support and collaboration hither-to received for the construction activities disintegrated at the imposition of many tongues.

Consequently, the building activity came to abrupt halt, and the tower was abandoned unfinished. The bewildered tower builders were helpless and unprepared to meet the communication crisis. The orderly transition from one common language to many languages, and the dissipation of the rank and file of the early postdiluvian age were a deathblow to the Babel conspiracy.

The Bible account indicates that every spoken human language is a result of that encounter at Babel. Therefore every one born of a woman is born into a pre-determined language group. We should see all the languages of the world today as a makeshift for a common language in the new world. There is however a pre-requisite and basic language for citizenship in the earth made new. Every prospective citizen for God's kingdom and theocracy in the new and sinless world ought to learn and speak the language of love here and now.

Hate Crime and the Christian

Every believing Christian and those whose hearts are inclined to the truth must reflect on the following words: "If anyone says, 'I love God', yet hates his brother, he is a liar. For anyone who does not love his brother whom he has seen, cannot love God whom he has not seen" (1 John 4:20). John does not speak of a biological brother. In the restricted usage brother refers to all believers who make up the Church of God, the one family of God. In its broader usage brother includes any member of the human race. The brotherhood and sisterhood of all the groups of the human race is biblically irrefutable (Acts 17:26). We are all by creation descendants of Adam and Eve. That brotherhood and sisterhood of all humanity is further established by common circumstances through the death and resurrection of Jesus. It is also confirmed by the redemption made available unto all men through the blood of Jesus (Isa. 53:2; 2 Cor. 5:14, 15; 1 Thess. 5:10).

The Bible indicates that ill feeling or hatred would cease where there is love (Rom. 13:10). What is love? This four-letter word means different things to many people. To begin with, love is one of the basic emotions resulting from psychological and physiological changes in the body. The arousal of love emotion, like every other emotion, depends not so much on a stimulus situation as on how the situation is preceived. In other words, motivation to love depends not so much on the object of our love as on how the object is perceived and valued. If the object of our love is perceived as a significant other or familiar and friendly, our love emotion is constantly aroused and sustained. A prayerful study of Apostle Paul's treatise on love (see 1 Cor. 13) leads to an understanding of the nature and meaning of love. Love is more than committing time, talents, and material wealth to helping others. It is more than donating all that one has for missionary work at home and abroad. Love is neither giving casually for the poor nor distributing religious literature to "none Christian lands". Love is not really what one does or gives in time of crises or at convenient time to one's kith and kin. Love is both a disposition of the heart and assent of the mind with unconditional acceptance of and friendship with fellow man irrespective of skin color, language, and ethnic background.

There is no justifiable basis for hate crimes against any colored person[1]. Humanity is created in different colors. Humankind has its minor differences in physical features. These differences in skin color, physical features, and languages are not meant to divide humankind into races. There is one and only one human race, because "there is one kind of flesh of men" (1 Cor. 15:39). Some ancient manuscript omits the phrase "of flesh" to have the passage read: "There is one kind of men." The Bible affirms a common origin of humankind. The evolutionist theorizes the beginning of all human life

---

1   The term "colored person" or "colored people" used in this book refers to every complexion. For the black, for example, a light or brown-yellow skin is considered colored, and vice versa.

from a common speck of life. Science too does not disprove the affirmation of the word of God. It supports and confirms the creationist's view and teaching that all men are made of the same substance. The common substance with which all men are made would invalidate and make the grouping of humanity into more than one race unscriptural. The differing human skin colors are not for incompatible existence among all the groups of the human race. In fact, the one ancestry and source of humankind, and the common fate that befalls humanity, would make hate a crime against humanity.

If viewed from the backdrop of the teachings of the Bible, all acts of hate, verbally expressed and implied in a look or otherwise, are symptoms. These symptoms are a reflection of warped thinking. An acknowledgment of God's perfect creation, and acceptance of the brotherhood of all color and language groups would make an aversion of human skin color or contempt of any language group a serious dysfunction of the heart and mind. We should admit the seriousness of our faulty thinking about other ethnic or color group. And earnestly seek for that transforming power of the Holy Spirit to clear our head of that negative stuff that often blur our perception of other people. It is not until we reach to a stage in our spiritual growth where we see and treat every one as creation of God and human life as sacred will our son-ship or daughter-ship be legitimatized in the family of God. Also until we outgrow our prejudices, biases, contempt and discrimination of persons who are different from us in color, language, and ethnic background, our claim to living truth and conversion is false and deceptive.

While it is hard to justify inter-racial hostility, it is harder to comprehend and justify intra-racial and ethnic conflicts in the world today. Of course, these raging conflicts validate the reliability of eschatological prophecies of the Christian Bible (2 Tim. 3:1–3; cf Rom. 1:28–32), and characterize a world in need of inner beauty and strength.

Prejudice: God speaks through Peter's Vision

In the days of the apostles, there was a class and racial distinction between the Jews and the non-Jews, the "Gentiles". This was a carry-over from the Old Testament era. The intervention of heaven became urgent and necessary because of the inhibiting nature of the practice to the growth and expansion of the gospel.

A vision was shown to Apostle Peter. In the vision, Peter saw the heaven open and a sheet descending. In the sheet were different kinds of wild and unclean beasts and birds. Peter was asked, three times, to kill and prepare for his meal the wild and unclean beasts and birds. But Peter refused at each instruction to kill and eat the unclean beasts and birds. It was against his Jewish practice and diet to eat what is considered unclean (Lev. 11:1–47). Peter's refusal was met with heaven's declaration: "What God hath cleansed that call not thou common" (Acts 10:11–15, KJV). The Jews rejected and isolated the non-Jews. Even the Jewish converts to the Christian religion could not outgrow this negative feeling and attitude towards their fellow Gentile converts. The vision of the four-footed beasts was in its entirety symbolic. It was designed to teach, firstly, that all humankind is a creation of God, and secondly, that no group of the human race should be regarded as unclean, common and inferior. The Apostle Peter did not, at first, understand what was shown to him. But the visit of the Gentiles, and the Holy Spirit's impression upon Peter to accept the Gentiles' invitation for a preacher, convinced him that the vision was symbolic. The four-footed and unclean beasts represent the Gentiles who were regarded and treated as inferior and common creatures. Peter affirmed, "God hath shown me that I should not call any man common or unclean" (Acts 10:28; cf., Matt. 5:22). At a later time when his fellow Jews questioned his authority for his ministry among the Gentiles, Peter rehearsed what was shown him in the vision, and asked, "Who was I that I could withstand God?" (Acts 11:17). Peter said, in other words, that it is an affront with God to refuse to recognize God's creation in the Gentiles. The evidence is clear and compelling in the vision. Peter admitted the absurdity of racial and class distinction between the Jews and the non-Jews. The fact that the Gentiles too deserve salvation of God is an undeniable evidence of inestimable value and worth of the non-Jews.

Those who take seriously the word of God for counsel and guidance should find Peter's vision informative and helpful in formulating a personal policy regarding their inter-racial and intra-racial relations.

Hostility or hatred against anyone for his/her skin color, language, or ethnic background is misplaced. No one but God should be held responsible for what man had no control over with. Neither should any man's skin color or racial and language group be the object of hate. Man had no choice over his skin color and racial group, as much as he has no choice over his gender. That's why a negative attitude and rejection of anyone for no reason other than the color or language is a disbelief and rejection of God's divine choice and gifts for man. The unconverted converts of the Christian religion and all those who either have an aversion for any human skin color or contemptuous of a language group would stand before God as murderers, and despisers of God's creation (1 John 3:15; Matt. 5: 21, 22).

Prejudice: God speaks through Miriam's Experience

Sacred record reveals that Zipporah, a black woman, was married to Moses, a Jew (Exod. 2:21; 3:1; 4:18, 20). The happily married Moses dwelt with his father-in-law for a time, until God asked him to return back to Egypt (Exod. 4:19). Moses left Midian with his wife, Zipporah, and their two sons. But on the way to Egypt, Moses sensed some hardship and unbearable situations for his wife and children. Consequently, he sent them back to his father-in-law in Midian. Later, on a visit to his son-in-law, Jethro with Zipporah and her two sons met with Moses at the camp in Rephidim. It was a happy family reunion for Moses and his wife, Zipporah and their two sons. The reunion was celebrated with a feast organized and hosted by Jethro. All the elders of Israel with Aaron attended the feast (Exod. 18:21). Not long after, Israel moved out of the camp in Rephidim, and pitched briefly from one location to another. When they came to Hazeroth Miriam and Aaron murmured against Moses, their sibling brother. That murmuring and opposition is recorded for the Christian Church today.

In the book of Numbers 12:1–15, we read that Miriam and Aaron spoke against Moses because of his marriage with Zipporah, an Ethiopian. Not only were Miriam and Aaron disappointed with Moses for his marriage to a black woman, they could not see themselves as subordinates to Moses. They bragged over the fact that they, too, had the prophetic gift, and direct communication with God. Moses, however, went about his daily duty without a word to Miriam and Aaron. He defended not his position and marriage, but left it with God to handle. And God did. He summoned Moses, Aaron and Miriam to appear before him. God reiterated the obvious facts. His relationship with Moses was intimate and special beyond and above his relationship with any other prophet or leader in Israel. God then demanded from Aaron and Miriam to show cause why they should not be punished for their boldness in criticizing Moses for his marriage with a black woman.

Without any doubt the marriage had received God's seal of approval. Also, Aaron and Miriam were arraigned before God for equating their position with Moses' position among the people. God who is both the plaintiff and the judge, found the murmuring brother and sister guilty. Consequently, Miriam alone was sentenced to a seven-day quarantine with leprosy. Probably, she was the chief instigator of the opposition against Moses. (Num. 12:10–15).

The place and timing of the murmuring and opposition against Moses have led to the assumption that Miriam had some personal grudges with Zipporah, her sister-in-law.

Recasting the dramatic text with related passages, the following points emerge:

1. There was a family feud.

2. The chief instigator of the feud was Miriam.

3. At the center or the cause of the feud was Zipporah.

4. Miriam had been popular with her people as a prophetess, song composer, singer, and choir director. She was, probably, the director for the women's ministry of the Church in the wilderness (Acts 7:38). By her position and gender she was consulted for issues that affected the women folk in the camp (Exod. 15:20).

5. The arrival of Zipporah, the first lady, brought some changes and reorganization in Miriam's consultation and counseling positions. Some consultations that were made to Miriam, and matters which hitherto had been within her portfolio, were now transferred to Zipporah.

6. Moses would no longer share his concerns, and burdens with Miriam, but would share them with Zipporah, a trusted wife who had proved her intelligence and love even in the time of crisis and emergencies (Exod. 4:18–26)

7. Zipporah was, probably, not in the limelight of the nation's political activities, but as a wife of a public and political figure she worked behind the scene to bring a desired change.

8. Her position as the first lady was challenging but nonetheless, coveted by many. Zipporah with her religious background and the discipline of motherhood had proved equal to the task. She worked consistently to maintain a positive influence over and beyond her immediate family circle. Thus, her rare quality of character and position must have earned her the admiration of all Israel, and the jealousy of Miriam.

9. Evidently, Zipporah's position and positive influences were unrecognized, unappreciated, and even discredited by Miriam. And Miriam's name-calling and references to Zipporah's skin color and racial group cannot be refuted.

10.   Miriam socially isolated Zipporah. Thus, for a time refused to consult with and receive orders or directives from Moses. And to cover up her prejudices and insubordinations, Miriam protested: "Has the Lord indeed spoken only through Moses? Has he not spoken through us also?" (Num. 12:2).

11. God's response and reaction was swift and drastic. He castigated Miriam and Aaron for equating Mosaic high office with their secondary and subordinate position and role. God reacted directly to Miriam's probable racist or ethnocentric remarks and insubordination. She was inflicted with leprosy, a dreadful and loathsome disease. By the health and sanitation law of the nation (Lev. 13:46; Num. 5:2, 3), Miriam, the Leper was isolated from the camp of Israel, and quarantined.

It was a just retribution for making Zipporah, the black woman, a social outcast of the family. Miriam was to learn from this experience the low self-esteem, emotional anguish and emptiness of an isolated and outcast of the society.

The following points are underscored as we conclude this chapter.

Reaction to human skin colors varies. Some people whole-heartedly accept and tolerate colored persons. Some openly tolerate but secretly anathematize a colored person. Still some are openly hostile to colored persons. In spite of some three differing human skin colors on the earth, there is only one human race. The one human race is established in creation and recreation. In creation mankind is formed and made of one substance. In recreation Jesus Christ offered his life for all. His death on the cross for all indicates that all men of whatever color are equal and worthy of salvation. Hostility or discriminatory act for one's skin color is a crime against God's creation, and a misplaced anger against the innocent.

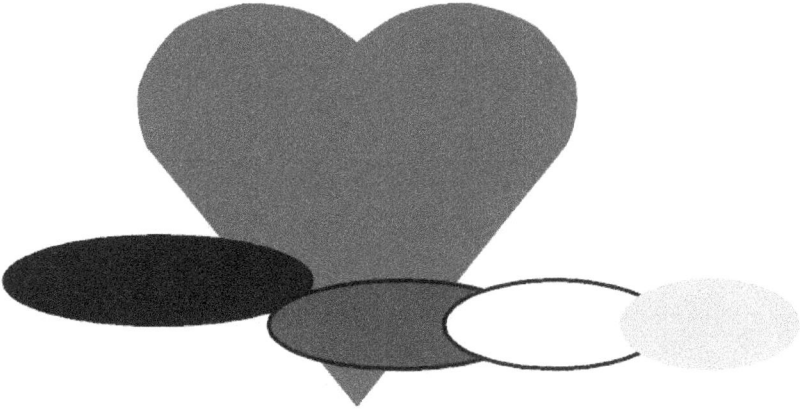

Love is color blind

At the Cross

Egocentrism and sectionalism are abhorred to shame
Tribalism and racism are nailed to rot
Biases and prejudices are pinned to rust
Color and language groups embrace to live
The Cross a melting pot for all colors and tongues
draws all men and women to fame

Some reaction to human skin color has been reviewed. A definition of love, and Biblical stand against hatred, prejudices, and the like has also been discussed.

The following chapter discusses some practical means of discrediting God and his perfect work in man. It presents a biblical concept of beauty, and points out some dangers with popular device and preparations for physical beauty.

Chapter 4

MAKEUP AND THE BIBLE

The objective of this chapter is to discuss all that is involved in the use of makeup. The General position of the Bible on makeup beauty or outward adornment is examined. This is followed by a discussion of the use of makeup in relation to time.

The Bible and Makeup

The book of Isaiah describes the makeup addict and beautician as "haughty, walking along with outstretched necks, flirting with their eyes tripping along with mincing steps, with ornaments jingling on their ankles" (Isa. 3:16). Apostle Paul writes to all Christians: "Do not offer the parts of your body to sin as instruments of wickedness, but rather offer yourselves to God, as those who have been brought from death to life; and offer the parts of your body to him as instruments of righteousness" (Rom. 6:13). This text speaks to many a man or woman who sees and uses his/her body as a means to an end that may dishonor God. One who makes idol of his/her body parts, an object of intense and passionate devotion with an intention of drawing undue attention for a selfish end. The use of any part of the body for what it is not intended is clearly implicated in the text. For example, the mouth and the anus are designed for and function as digestive tracts. But what do we see today? The mouth and anus are turned into and used as organs for sexual intercourse. These organs are turned into instruments of disobedience to natural law because anal intercourse and oral-genital activity are an abuse and misuse of the body. The word of God describes the unnatural use of the body as "vile passions, shameful, an error, and unfitting" for man (Rom. 1:26–28 NKJV).

45

Also implicated in the text are gang related tattoos, and piercing of body parts for ornaments. We do not judge the motivations for tattoos and /or pierced body parts. However, one wonders the place and eternal value of the tattoos, pierced and ornamented body parts in the praise and worship of God. After all God through Moses legislated against tattoos. Tattoos are associated with pagan rites, and idolatry (Lev. 19:28).

Further, the Bible text does not spare beauty preparations. The use of makeup has turned human body into a shrine for the goddess of beauty. As a matter of fact the Bible presents no good picture for makeup.

Some instances where cosmetics or makeup were used or mentioned indicate a sad end. For example, Jezebel painted her eyes and plaited her hair to look beautiful and attractive. When she looked out of the window she was attracted to Jehu, the recently anointed king of Israel. That look and attraction ended in the execution of the attractive Jezebel (2 Kings 9:30–33). Israel is likened to a woman who adorned herself with cosmetics, and whose makeup beauty could not save from destruction (Jer. 4:30).

The Bible cautions, "Your beauty should not come from outward adornment. Instead it should be that of your inner self, the unfading beauty of a gentle and quiet spirit, which is of great worth in God's sight" (1 Pet. 3:3, 4). The Bible speaks of two types of beauty. The physical beauty, that which is super-imposed by outward adornment. The second is the beauty that develops from within, springs up and radiates outwardly, a gentle and quiet spirit. A Christian virtue that reflects the serenity of heaven and elicits enduring joy and smile to those who court and embrace it. Gentle and quiet spirit is a moral beauty that does not depreciate in value and public admiration in old age, sickness or material poverty. It is the beauty of inner self that attracts heaven to earth, and lifts the earth up to heaven. Physical and outward beauty not backed up by beauty of moral character is worthless.

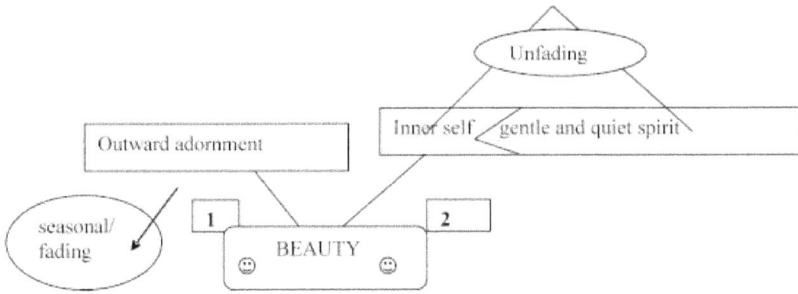

Two types of beauty (1 Pet. 3:3, 4)

Our society today seeks a comely body. A cosmetic procedure called *microdermabrasion* is gaining popularity among, mostly, women. The procedure works to remove the top layer of the skin, exposing the inner layer for growth of a healthy, radiant skin. Microdermabrasion is claimed to help promote healthy, young-looking skin. Middle aged and older women who want to look younger than their age are lured to it. They see the procedure their best bet to defy aging signs on their physical appearance. Let us come to terms with reality. dermatologists know that skin cells proliferate throughout human life. Also the skin cells are designed to timely replace dead or damaged tissue, retaining the authentic pigment of the skin.

The cosmetic procedure that removes, prematurely, the outer layer of the skin assumes the natural functions of the skin cells. Besides, removing the outer layer that protects, exposing the inner layer of the skin is reversing the order of nature. The abrading effect of microdermabrasion is nothing short of skinning a living human to satisfy the sensual. The glowing and younger-looking skin effect of the cosmetic procedure should be likened to a chemically de-greened fruits. Fruits, such as tomatoes may be prematurely ripened with chemicals to look reddish and fresh. Evidently, chemically ripened fruits may have long-term toxic effect on the human body. The beauty therapist or dermatologist sees microdermabrasion an answer to or solution for "a healthy younger-looking skin" that defies human aging. But the fact is that the wear and tear of life common with all humans makes aging process irreversible. The "radiant younger-looking skin" for life is a gift and reward for all citizens of a recreated world (Isa. 65:20, 22; 1 Cor. 15:51–53; Rev. 22: 1, 2). It cannot be realized in a sin-infested and diseased world of ours. By the way, a passionate devotion to physical beauty is intimated in the Scriptures as a characteristic of the end time professed Christians (Jude 8, 17–19; 2 Tim. 3:1–5). In some Christian homes prayer has been replaced with a daily ritual honoring the physical body with tubes of various colors for the face, eyes, and lips. In fact the ritual is proudly and openly performed on the air, land, and seas, suggesting space is no limit for displaying cosmetic beauty.

The Bible likens a name (character) to a pleasing fragrance of a perfume. Comparing a perfume/cosmetics with a name(character), the Bible recommends a good name/character a better choice, and "more desirable than great riches" (Eccles. 7:1; Song of Sol. 1:3; Prov. 22:1).

It is the moral character, man's indispensable inward beauty that endures even beyond the grave. The Apostle John wrote, "Blessed are the dead who die in the Lord from henceforth. Yea, saith the Spirit that they may rest from their labors, and their *works* do follow them" (Rev. 14:13, KJV). Men and women are remembered for their character, services or contributions to the society. It is the quality of character that endears or demeans a person before friends and foes.

The general characteristics of makeup, its source and ultimate end are described in the word of God: "For all that is in the world, the lust of the flesh, lust of the eyes, and the pride of life is not of the father, but is of this world. The world with its lust passes away, but he that doeth the will of God abides forever" (1 John 2:16, 17, KJV). What we need today is a spiritual bleaching and toning of the heart. The heart is the part of the body that is seen only by God. The state or condition of the heart can produce lasting joy and healing to the whole body, or eternal sorrow and destruction to body and soul. God's counsel to every one should not be overlooked: "Circumcise yourself to the Lord and take away the foreskin of your heart" (Deut. 10:16; Jer. 4:4). "Because out of the heart proceeds evil thoughts, murders, adulteries and fornication... (Matt.15:19, NKJV). To circumcise the heart means to rid the heart of impure thoughts, selfishness, and immorality. The beauty of the heart transcends the physical or facial beauty.

The Implications of the use of makeup

Suppose you have a flower vase in your home. And suppose you woke up one morning to hear the flower vase questioning, "Why did you make me into a brown or red vase?" How would you feel? Insulted? Yes, of course. But what will you do? Perhaps, break the vase into countless pieces, or remold it into another shape and color? Whatever may be your decision or reaction to the question posed by the vase, it is clear that your intelligence or wisdom has been questioned and doubted. Also, your good intention and purpose for the flower vase is despised and unappreciated.

We in effect question God's intelligence and wisdom when we use bleaching creams for a lighter skin color. The use of makeup in the pretext of looking beautiful and attractive is by implication a discontentment with the skin color given us by God. To deface and make up the skin is an affront with God. In response to that discontentment, God questioned, "Shall what is formed say to him who formed it, 'Why did you make me like this?'" (Isa. 45:9; Rom. 9: 20). This question should not be taken lightly or dismissed with a wave of the hand. God calls us to reflect on his creation to know who and what we are. Does the human body need any makeup or bleaching creams? That, perhaps, would be acceptable if the human body was a product of evolution. But to those who believe and accept as the truth the biblical account of creation, the human body is made, seen and declared by God as "very good" (Gen. 1:31).

Besides, God, through the prophet Isaiah, declares, "Everyone who is called by my name for I have created him for my glory, I have formed him; yea, I have made him" (Isa. 43:7, KJV). God chose three action words—*created, formed, and made*—to highlight, first, the originality of His product, man; and secondly, His divine and personal touch that produced a living being who is perfect in form or structure and in color. And thirdly, God takes the credit and full responsibility and with satisfaction for that product when He asserts, "I have made him." The work is done and complete. God was extremely careful and detailed in the plan to make man, and in its execution. Man is God's workmanship and the masterpiece of His creation (Eph. 2:10). Man is meticulously made beyond human comprehension (Ps. 139:14). Human body should not be treated as an unfinished piece of work that needs backup and makeup. The use of makeup and body bleaching devices is by implication an attempt to recreate and improve upon the physical appearance. Thus, a denial of God's claim and right upon the human body. We should know that in the spiritual realm it is impossible to change our sinful nature by external measure (Jer. 2:22; 13:23). So it is in the natural realm. It is impossible for a leopard to change its spots, as it is for human skin color to change. The futility of an attempt to bring a change through an external device is beautifully and fittingly described in these words: "Though you grind a fool in a mortar, grinding him like grain with a pestle, you will not remove the folly from him" (Prov. 27:22).

Many people often ask, "What is wrong with the use of makeup and body bleaching preparations?" My response comes with a question, "What is wrong with the natural skin color we are born with?" Surprisingly, my response is further met with another question, "What is wrong with making the natural skin color look beautiful and attractive with some makeup?"

Human body is the temple of God (1 Cor. 3:16; 6:19; 2 Cor. 6:16). Temple is a place dedicated for worship and holy services. The body temple is a dwelling place for the Spirit. It is sanctified for the glory of God. The human body is also pictured as vessel, sanctified unto God's honor. The use of makeup glorifies not God but the self. It makes a toy of God's temple. The indwelling Spirit of God is, certainly, not attracted to where self reigns supreme.

Do you give a thought to why people are always advised to stop the use of makeup, alcoholic liquor, and smoking when they are preparing or scheduled for major surgery? Evidently, makeup, alcoholic liquor, and smoking are a risk to one's health. In most cases they lead to operational or surgical complications, and hinder or delay the healing process. The makeup, in particular, causes skin coloration, which may lead to skin tear at the touch of the surgeon's staples. Apart from the potential harmful effect of the chemical contents of the cosmetics upon the user, the use of makeup or skin lightener for beauty and attraction is a fake, and a deception. We need to be very careful of the claims for the use of makeup. Those with low self-esteem and lack of self-confidence are easily enticed to wearing makeup as a means of attracting attention and improving their self-image. To use makeup as a cover-up for emotional insecurity or as a nonverbal expression of a desire for acceptance is a denial of reality. It is seeking for a healing with something that has no healing property in it. In the words of an Angel of God, it is like "seeking the living among the dead" (Luke 24:5). It is re-living the experience of the women followers of Jesus who went looking for the risen and living Jesus among the dead in the grave. The result of their search was disappointing until they were redirected to the right place where the living Jesus was to be found.

The low self-esteem is a state of the mind. It is not a spot or disease of the skin which could be cured by changing or improving the physical appearance of the body with makeup. The low self-esteem is more of a relational need or problem than of a physical look and appearance. Therefore, the right and tested step to gaining self-confidence and improving self-esteem is turning to a trusted and proven friend, one who believes in you and appreciates your human worth. The only friend who loves at all times, in spite of what man is and regardless of man's inclination toward evil, is Jesus. His genuine love was revealed when he died in man's stead (Prov. 17:17; John 15:13). But friendship with Jesus is an active relationship, which involves the mind, the heart, and the hands. First, the human mind must be drawn and focused unto Jesus. The mind is the powerhouse of the body. Who or what controls the mind controls the man. When the mind is surrendered and united with the mind of Jesus by daily feeding on the eternal or spiritual food which he offers, there is a change that is wrought from within. Man's thought for his fellows would reflect God's thought. God's thought for man is a thought of good and not evil (Isa. 55:8, 9; Ps. 139:17). Besides, man would recognize his true nature, and see him/herself as an instrument or vessel of honor unto the creator God. There is a healing and peace with a total and full surrender of the mind to a trusted friend (Isa. 26:3). Secondly, friendship with Jesus involves the heart. The heart is the seat of affection. Therefore, it must be purified of self-centeredness. And be filled with the desire to reach and touch other lives. Thirdly, active participation and involvement in the work of improving the quality of man's social and moral life is an integral part of a meaningful relationship with Jesus. Your hands must be the hands of Jesus that ministered healing to a leper, the untouchable and outcast of the society who needed emotional as much as physical healing (Matt. 8:3; Mark 1:4; Luke 5:12). This active involvement in the lives of others brings emotional healing and improves self-esteem.

A terminally ill Christian woman was told she has a couple of months to live. What do you think she did? Spent her days in beauty salon? Or cursing and brooding over her unfortunate situation? She was neither an evolutionist nor a die-hard atheist. She spent the days mending breached relationships with her God, and neighbors by prayers and visitations. Eventually, she cheated and beat a cancerous death for eleven years. What has happened? Was it a miracle or sheer luck? Whatever it was, her daily communication with God in His Word and prayer, and devotion to others with loving deeds were an undeniable factor that affected and changed her life. The less she thought of self and more of others, she received a healing miracle of grace.

If beauty of inner self (see diagram in page 47) is a gentle and quiet disposition then the low self-esteem or the ugliest of the world can be the most beautiful through unbroken connection with Jesus. Jesus invites everyone to "come…take my yoke upon you and learn from me for I am gentle and humble in heart" (Matt. 11:28, 29).

Jesus indicates that his yoke is an aid to learning his gentle and humble character. The Apostle Peter sees gentleness and humility as unfading beauty. What is this yoke that reveals the beauty and the best in Jesus? Like every yoke Christ's yoke binds to service.

The yoke that binds to service is the law of love for God and man. Jesus shunned all pomp and display. He was actively engaged in the ministry and service of love for all humanity. The gospel writers present Jesus as a man consumed with a passion for selfless service all the days of his life on earth .He revealed by his exemplary life that the secret for priceless beauty and self-esteem is in taking the yoke that binds to service.

Also, an important step to improving self-esteem is not found in the claims of the dietician and the fashion designer. For example, the dietician claims, "You are what you eat." The fashion designer asserts, "You are what you wear." But the Scriptures would say, "You are what you think" (Prov. 23:7, KJV). Evidently, what you think you are influences what you eat and wear. It influences your behavior or action. Therefore, positive thinking of yourself as a complete and physically perfect creation of God will do what the ingredients of makeup are incapable of achieving in your life

There are those who wear makeup to either enhance their physical appearance or to look feminine. It is not so much the external as the internal factor that enhances the physical look and personality. When the effort to "improve" the physical appearance to the neglect of the inner self, it is like renovating the exterior wall of a building when its soiled rooms are not cared for. Certainly, there is no joy at the sight of those annoying and stubborn little roaches left to crawl freely around the unkempt rooms.

Some married women, either encouraged by their husbands or by personal choice, wear makeup to appear attractive to their male partners and keep the marital relationship. The marital union established on that which conduces to outward beauty and sensuous attraction and base passion is fragile. The home is not built on the outward appearance of the spouses. It is the beauty of character that makes for eternal joy and peace at home. It is the beauty of my wife's character, for example, that attracts me back home when I am away. I feel at home because she is home.

Looking at the whole question of beauty, I have no problem believing that beauty is a creation of God. He is the source of beauty. God declared His creation, generally, beautiful. There is beauty all around us. Perhaps, no age recognizes and accepts more than this age a well-known saying, "A thing of beauty is a joy forever." Beauty is also a gift of God. Some look naturally and physically more beautiful or handsome than their fellows. That-not-withstanding, no one would disagree with the fact that acceptance and admiration are some basic emotional or psychological needs of humankind. Naturally, all of us want to be accepted and admired by others, at least, for what we are. Some, however, want acceptance and admiration for their look. Their pre-occupation is to appear outwardly beautiful and/or "sexy" with makeup and makeover. But the beauty that concerns us most, and which is an enduring source of joy, is the moral character. It is a beauty that is developed, nursed, and nurtured with no monetary cost. Besides, many have discovered that "all that glitters is not gold." That physical beauty and makeup or cosmetic beauties are not sustainable source of joy. It is hard to court long, engage and wed with physical beauty that is bereft of moral conduct. You see, what matters here and now is who we are inside out. But, regrettably, many a Christian who represents the interest and values of heaven before the world has become a key participant in the race for comely beauty. When the Christian appears focused to the sky of eternal beauty, while his/her mind and soul is wrapped up with the fading dross of earthly beauty, it is hypocrisy. The witnessing power of the Christian to the world is weakened and invalidated. There may not be anything sinful and evil about wearing makeup. However, the implications, the thinking, and the motivations behind its use raise the question, "Is man better off with the use of makeup or worse off without its use?"

Influence of Dualism

Perhaps, the undue attention given to physical and outward appearance today is a reaction against the excesses of the age of "soul beauty". The Greek philosophy of dualism dichotomized man into "soul" and "body" or "spirit" and "flesh". The acceptance of the Greek world-view by the Church influenced the theology, lifestyle, and practices of the religious world. The "soul" and the "body" were seen and taught as two independent identities. Each was treated in isolation of the other. The body was regarded as a "house" in which the all-important and immortal soul has a temporary abode. Some view and liken the body to a prison house for the soul. They claim that the incarcerated soul is eventually released when the mortal body dies. Besides, the body is thought to be matter and sinful which should not be nursed or aided to corrupt the soul. Thus, the body was abused, exposed to extreme heat and/or cold, lacerated, and denied of raiment and food. During the days of the Apostle Paul, and in the Roman world, some religious leaders advocated and promoted an ascetic lifestyle. They believe it to be a religious means of attaining the highest spirituality and wisdom. But Apostle Paul countered, "Such relations indeed have an appearance of wisdom, with their imposed worship, their false humility and their harsh treatment of the body, but they lack any value in restraining sensual indulgence" (Col. 2:20–23; 1 Tim. 4:1–3).

Furthermore, asceticism and celibacy were both regarded by the Church as virtue, and a religious lifestyle that would keep the "soul" or "spirit" pure and undefiled. The ascetic and the celibate were taught and encouraged to shun every luxury and pleasure of the body or flesh in order to focus completely on the spiritual things. For this end, marriage was viewed as a worldly concern. The expression of intimacy in sex was regarded as a fleshly lust, which dwarfs or inhibits the soul from attaining the spiritual goal. Recently a Church leader endorses the notion that the human body is a by-product of evolution process. He claims that a person's "spirit" and "dignity" are not subject to evolution process. The endorsement is a modern religious re-echo of the voice of dualism, and a belief in the superiority of the soul over the body or flesh. This brand of Christianity that endorses a theory that questions and doubts the literal word of God and its account of creation is up for a spiritual declension with a negative impact upon the world. The opposite effects of that endorsement which the Church and its leadership least anticipated is evident in the enthronement of the "seen" over the "unseen" and the "external" over the "internal".

Today, conscious reaction against the age of "soul beauty" is evident. The reaction mounts, and like the surging waters, it is sweeping away the vestige of the age of soul beauty. We live in an age of fashion where the body is adorned and adored. Physical beauty has taken the place of the inner beauty, and has become the all-consuming passion and the goal of many professed Christians. The makeup has been enthroned in the heart and thinking of men and women, both young and old, as the goddess of physical beauty. There is no part of the body that has been spared of the makeup touch. In the extreme, man is seen and treated as "all body and flesh" without a soul.

An undistorted perception of who we are, where we come from, and what human existence is all about, would reject the concept of dualism and the resultant treatment of man. The human body is neither the product of evolution nor a "house" for the soul, which needs constant renovation or remodeling with the makeup. It should be noted here that the human body/flesh is not an entity independent of the soul/spirit. When the body that was formed from the dust/clay of the ground became animated with the breath of life, the Bible says, "Man became a living soul" (Gen. 2:7, KJV). The man does not have a soul. In reality, the man is the living soul. The man/soul can sin, and is subject to destruction (Ezek. 18:4; Matt. 10:28). In a sense, the terms "body" and "spirit" should be likened to the two sides of a coin. You cannot disengage one side without ruining the wholeness of the coin. And if there is a deep scratch on one side, the coin in its totality is damaged. What affects the physical body of the man/soul would affect the spiritual realm of the man/soul. Therefore, both the concept of dualism and the use of makeup are based on a perverse view of man. They are a distortion of the meaning of human existence.

Besides, the humanist-evolutionist's belief in man's innate ability and capacity for self-change and perfection is also implied and reflected in the use of makeup. By implication makeup is man's attempt to make a change and improve his/her form and structure. This undue attention to the outward appearance makes one a slave to his/her own body. It is a conscious and unconscious belief that man lives unto the self and for the self. This is a form of idolatry.

The Christian and Makeup

A guest sat at a strategic spot with a clear view of every worshiper in the sanctuary. He takes notice of every movement and every look. He hears every whisper, and sees every gestures. In the middle of the worship hour, a worshiper with a glossy face, painted lips, manicured nails with shaded eyelids and brow walked in, tip toed all the way from the balcony to the front seat. Within minutes Rosemary attracted the attention of every worshiper. She clears her throat, and turns her eyes in every direction. At the end of the worship, the unknown visitor walked straight to Rosemary and asked: "May I know who you are"? Rosemary who had expected a compliment of admiration from the visitor responded: "I am Rosemary, a regular member of the Church" The visitor mused, and said: "I believe God formed Rosemary with no artificial features" "Yes, you are right", Rosemary admitted. "I am a makeup woman," she added. "No, the stranger countered, you made a masquerade of your real self." Rosemary could not be better described and characterized with her makeup.

Many Christians may use makeup as a lifestyle of modern living. For them it is fun, fashionable and sociable to wear makeup. They may be guided by clear conscience and motivated by a desire to be identical with others. But in no time and circumstance will "clear conscience" and "right motive" justify the use of makeup by the Christians when nothing of value and eternal worth is gained. It is unsafe to rest our argument in favor of a particular lifestyle or action on clear conscience or right motive. Conscience does not determine that which is right or wrong. Conscience acts and reacts from what is constantly fed to it. For example, a teenage boy who is fed constantly with infightings in the Church would grow into adulthood believing in altercations as a Christian way of life.

He would with a clear conscience and with no guilty feeling disrespect and fight with ordained ministers and/or fellow members of the Church. Similarly, a teenage girl who daily sees her mother drink, smoke, curse, and nag, would regard drinking and smoking, cursing and nagging as a normal lifestyle. The Bible indicates that man's conscience can be seared, weakened, and defiled (1 Tim. 4:2; Titus 1:15; 1 Cor. 8:10, 12).

The Christian, however, has the freedom to do that, which does not in any way violate God's moral law. But if the exercise of his liberty would lead one to err, the Bible warns, "Take heed lest by any means this liberty of yours become a stumbling block to them that are weak..." Paul adds, "Wherefore if meat (food) makes my brother to offend, I will eat no flesh while the world standeth, lest I make my brother to offend" (1 Cor. 8:9, 13; Rom. 14: 13–17, KJV). The limitation placed on the Christian's freedom (1 Cor. 10:28–33), and the principle guiding our action or freedom as it affects others should be applied to the question of whether or not to use makeup[1]. Freedom is no freedom without the responsibility and accountability to others who may be affected by our choices or actions. No one lives with out touching other lives.

Besides, the Bible recognizes the unique position of the Christian Church in the world. It characterizes the Christians, the spiritual Israel, as "peculiar nation" (1 Pet. 2:9; Titus 2:14; Deut. 14:2; Ps. 135:4). The Christian is in the world but not of the world (John 17:15, 16). The Christian is to be transformed and be conformed to the image of Jesus Christ (Rom. 8:29; 12:2). The transformed Christian stands out in

---

1   The use of makeup by one and its negative effects upon others, particularly, the non-users, is discussed in Chapter five of this work. There is no doubt that "private life or personal choice" may have a public consequence.

the world for Jesus. If the Christian conforms to the lifestyle of the unbelieving community, which he is called upon to bring to the saving knowledge of Jesus, his "peculiar" nature is lost. The Christian becomes powerless to effectively witness for the Lord.

Furthermore, heaven and the world respectively operate on different principles and priorities. The world, for example, adores the makeup body. It looks at and glorifies the outward appearance. But heaven looks at the heart, and glorifies the inner beauty. The Christian, therefore, must hold to the values of heaven, project and represent the interest of heaven to the world.

The acceptance of a standard and style that glorifies the self is a sale out of the Christian's birthright for that which perishes with time. To be identical with the world in order to win the world is playing a dangerous game with the Devil. The Christian should always be heaven-minded in order to draw the world heavenward. For what purpose does the Christian need makeup, or skin lighteners, age defying and wrinkle free creams? Has the Christian lost sight of a better world and a glorified body which will no longer be subject to decay? Makeup and other beauty preparations should be considered useless in the light of heaven's gift of immortal body.

Actors and actresses may have a genuine reason for the use of makeup if it is worn to protect the skin from the blanching effects of the light (Herman Buchman, "Makeup", *Encyclopedia Americana*, international edition, Vol. 18, Danbury, CT: Grolier Inc., 2000, 149). Do non-actors and non-actresses also use makeup to protect their skin from the stage light? In reality every Christian who wears a makeup is an actor or actress. Imagine three in every five women or one in every five men on the streets, in the churches, mosque, synagogues or temple, offices, and business houses wearing makeup. Evidently, the streets, religious worship centers, business homes and offices have been literally turned into theaters or Hollywood with professed Christians as actors and actresses. Do people "tune in" to the Church because they are impressed with our look, and not with who and what we represent? Jesus our model is despised when we wear makeup and make-over. "He had no (outward) beauty or majesty to attract us to him (and) nothing in His appearance that we should desire him" (Isa. 53:2). Not because he despised beauty.

There must, first, be stripes and lacerated body at the cross before a "glorious" body at the resurrection. A Bible writer recalls the effect of the beatings and says: "His appearance was so disfigured beyond that of any man and his form marred beyond human likeness" (Isa. 52:14). Regrettably, today, Christians seek after comely body when a homely but bled body of their Savior needs of them a soothing balm of self-denial.

The undue attention to outward beauty when the world is on its last course for demise or disintegration is a mistake. It may be costly and deadly to the Christian.

Makeup Lifestyle and Life's deadline

The philosopher speaks of "a time to be born and a time to die" (Eccles. 3:2). There is the beginning and the ending of life. Life is the interval between the day of birth and the day of death. Our thoughts, motivations, and what we do or how we live, are weighted contents of the timeline of our human existence. Job, the ancient sage of Luz complains: "Man's days are determined. You (God) have decreed the number of his months and have set limit he (man) cannot exceed" (Job 14:5). This is an unambiguous statement of God's deadline for man's existence within the bounds of time.

In view of the deadline, we need to know what life is all about. Our comprehension of the purpose of life would help us evaluate things, and make intelligent choice or decision.

Most Christians have no problem believing that we are created by God for His glory. But the life some live is very troubling, and reflects, if you please, a neonatal understanding of the purpose of life. Like the fool in Christ's parable, many do say: "Take life easy; eat, drink and be merry" (Luke 12:19). To such men and women life is a matter of socializing, eating and drinking. Life is measured by how much of the cosmetics worn, and the "quality time" with the opposite sexes. We play the arrogant fool with no serious reflection on our mortal nature. Cosmetics lifestyle either ignores or gives the spiritual and eternal a secondary place. The lifestyle is a "here-and-now" existence with no future.

Serious objection to cosmetics lifestyle includes: its appeal to, and preoccupation with physical attraction and beauty. The self is projected, and cosmetics are glorified. Cosmetics lifestyle is nothing short of selfism. God is left out. A relationship of discontent and disregard for God's work replaces accountability to God for the stewardship of time and our body. The truth is that we exist in time with a dead line.

How we live and what we live for must be in reference to the One who lives in time, before time, and beyond time, and in whose divine existence our human life has meaning and purpose. The quality of life is expressed in relationships. Therefore, it is not living in error, but the abuse and misuse of the time given to know and live out the truth that would disqualify any one from the eternal bliss with God in the coming recreated world.

Regrettably, we have accepted the "here-and-now" philosophy of life. We are merely dragging along the "here-and-now" animal existence with no consciousness for the future, and the deadline imposed upon us mortal beings. This here-and-now existence strongly influences our attitude towards time, in particular, and life in general. We see life for what it is here, and for what we can get out of it now. There is no conscious reflection of life's ultimate end and accountability tomorrow. The concern of many is centered on their outward appearance and physical beauty. We have become slaves and addicted to the makeup. We are glued to the dressing mirror fixing up the outer self twenty-four hours daily. We hardly relax to reflect on what life is in relation to time. Perhaps, Moses saw this lack of self-reflection, and the "here-and-now" philosophy among his own people. He pleads with God to: "Teach us to number our days aright, that we may gain a heart of wisdom", "Show me O Lord, my life's end and the number of my days; let me know how fleeting is my life" (Ps. 90:12; 39:4).

If one half of the time we spend standing before the dressing mirror or beauty salon for our outward appearance is spent in sober reflection of the meaning and purpose for our existence, the homes and the society would be better, safer, and immoral-free environment to live. There would be time for meaningful communications between spouses, and between parents and their children. In fact the focus would be shifted from the self to others and from the fleeting material things of the world to the enduring things of the heavenly.

Man is made to stand upright and to aim towards a higher, peaceful and death-free altitude. Therefore, we are to live beyond the present and into the future. The "here-and-now" philosophy of existence denies the fact that man is both a present-and future-oriented creature. We scarcely begin the present before the future sets in. If life is lived for here and now, and with no reference to the future consequences of the present, then the past will stand to witness against us for the failure to learn from it. The reliable guide and teachings of the past are with us today. The unfolding reality of life leads no one to doubt that "All flesh is grass, and all its beauty and glory is like the flower of the field that blossoms today and withers tomorrow" (Isa. 40:6–8).

There is a "living beauty" whose fragrance and attractions are sustained with time. There is a beauty, a "makeup beauty" whose fragrance is short-lived and gone at the wake of time. The makeup beauty is "flesh-borne" and skin deep because its composite material works only on the external and temporal. It does not stand the test of time. The makeup beauty is for here and now, and cannot be carried from beyond the present into the future.

The Christian who lives in the present and with reference to the past and the future would be wise to spend time with that which endures beyond the present. Because the One who has graciously put the skin colors in place cannot justify the time, and the money spent on the non-essential, and the fading shadows of life. That One has set up in no distant time, a tomorrow of reckoning and accountability for the stewardship of our body. "God will bring every deed into judgment, including every hidden thing, whether it is good or evil" (Eccles. 11:9, 10; 12:14; Heb. 9:27).

Motivations for the use of makeup may vary from person to person. But beneath the liberal use of makeup is a motivation for attention to the self, and allurement into sexual act. There is a close correlation between the use of makeup and the sexual act. The chapter that follows discusses the human sexuality in relation to the use of makeup.

All in the Cross

*The sacrifice on the cross could not be more real than
the oozing bloody water from His pierced body
Neither is the rejected vinegar incontrovertible reality
than the pain of the bleeding body
It is neither the vinegar nor the sight of a mother but
Believers' living faith in the dying son of God that
eased the harassing pain of the cross
He took our place with a homely and lacerated body
And gave us in his stead a resurrection morning of
a makeover head-to-toe
What more do we need that the cross has not provided?
Beauty? The cross is a model of beauty of character
Love? The cross lifts up a Savior who lives to love
Agelessness? A thirst for all that the cross stands for
and a daily walk in focus of the cross bring eternity
now and hereafter*

Chapter V

HUMAN SEXUALITY AND MAKEUP

This chapter discusses human sexuality. The contextual frame and meaning of sexual acts are examined. This is with the view of underscoring the insidious and corrupting influences of makeup lifestyle on human sexuality and morality.

Makeup and Sex

Some lewd men and women evidently use makeup to their advantage. They turn to makeup as an unsuspected device for enticement. The captivating power of makeup, and the enticing effects of the flashy made up body ultimately leads many a man and a woman into sexual immorality. For many, sex has become a commodity and/or source of pleasure. Thus, the use of makeup for sex questions the conservative concept and stand for human sexuality. It also supports the liberal view of sex for all, and, exclusively, for pleasure. The subject of human sexuality must, therefore, be approached objectively. It must be seen and defined for what and whom it is made.

Human Sexuality

Human sexuality is a subject least understood, most abused and misused for what it is not. The computer/technology age with television, in particular, has glamorized and commercialized sex to the point of treating it like an open park where pleasure seekers can freely spend their recreation time. For many, sex has become an article of exchange for money and position. There is, however, a better way of looking at sex that befits the dignity of man as rational and responsible being.

What is sex? To give an accurate answer to the question, we need to know, first, the social and ethical context of human sexuality. The context and objective way of looking at sex are in relation to the institution that gives it its legality and humanness, and which makes human sexuality different from the sex life of the beast or the like. The institution is marriage.

Marriage was instituted in the Garden of Eden in the Near East more than six thousand years ago. From the viewpoint of the One who instituted it, and united the first couple in holy wedlock, marriage is a covenant of life-long dependence and inter-dependence between a man and a woman. It is a covenant of living, sharing, and growing together.

And for some cultural groups, marriage is a bond between the male and the female and their respective families.

Every covenant is made in confidence of the covenanters. And because of its relational nature, covenant is ratified to confirm or assure its validity or authenticity. Among some ancient peoples of the world, agreements of a major or life and death consequence were sealed with blood.

The Bible presents instances where God entered into covenant relationship with, first, individuals who represent the human race—Adam, Noah, and Abraham—(Gen. 2:16; 3:15; 9:16; 12:2), and secondly, the ancient Israel (Exod. 19:4–8; 24:3–8). Also, the Bible presents a "new covenant" between God and "spiritual Israel", God's chosen people from the entire human race (Heb. 8:6–13; 9:1–22). These covenants were ratified with blood, the life-giving fluid. God's covenant relationship with the entire human race, for example, was ratified with the shed blood of Jesus. The blood shows the importance of the agreement, and its life-long binding claims upon the parties.

Marriage covenant between a man and a woman, under normal or healthy circumstance, is ratified by the two. This is done not by an exchange of wedding rings or by the officiating minister declaring the newlyweds as husband and wife. Marriage is, symbolically, ratified when the man literally gives himself to the woman and the woman willingly and literally gives up herself to the man in sexual intercourse. The man and the woman seal and ratify by sexual act their marital vows to bear the responsibility of living together for life. Sexual intimacy is a symbol of sealing and/or renewal of that life-long commitment for oneness. A seal is placed on a done deal. An agreement is ratified only after it has been made. Marriage, therefore, precedes sexual intercourse. Sexual intimacy should also be seen as a sealing of that life-long commitment for oneness. Sex before or outside marriage is an irresponsible act. It makes a mockery of God's institution of marriage. Any device or preparation that encourages that irresponsible behavior should not be used or promoted by any Christian.

An incident recorded in the Bible illustrates the significance of and the obligation imposed upon sexual intimacy. The Bible reveals that Amnon seduced and raped his half-sister, Tamar. He did not want to accept responsibility for his action by refusing to marry her, even though such marriage was acceptable by the society at that time. Tamar protested, "No, sending me away would be a greater wrong than what you have done to me" (2 Sam. 13:12–16). Tamar's protest before and after she was raped and refused in marriage testifies to the fact that sex must be within the realm and context of marriage.

To renounce the responsibility of marrying the sex partner, and/or to break away from the legal marital relationship after any sexual intercourse is condemned as an evil greater and treacherous than the premarital or extra-marital sex.

A Belief about Sex

An observation is made that in olden days, boys and girls matured late, but were married soon after their maturity. But in our own time and age, boys and girls mature early because of improved medical services, proper dieting, and improved standards of living. Also their reproductive organs develop and are ready early. These children are expected to remain unmarried until after years of academic preparations, and with a reliable source of income. The observer then asked, "Why should the Church want these sexually mature boys and girls 'burn' through the years without sex until they get married? What will the society think of a mother who refuses to feed her baby when the baby cries for food? Will the woman not be accused of abuse and endangering the life of her child?"

The observer's question is borne out of the thinking and belief that sexual desire is no different from hunger or thirst. Let's consider first the question of the nursing mother with her baby. A wise mother plans for her baby's feeding schedule. The woman knows the right food and the right time to feed the baby. The baby's cry does not dictate or determine its feeding schedule. Following the schedule, though not rigidly, is a valuable training for the child to develop self-control.

Like the baby whose feeding is not denied but regulated by a wise and experienced mother, the sexually mature youth is not denied sexual expression. But the expression must be within its right and legal context. The Creator God who knows what is best for His creation has established a blueprint for man's sexual life. The sexually mature youth is under an obligation to exercise self-control, and remain a virgin until he/she gets married. The state of virginity has no serious and negative effect on the personality or physical and emotional development of the youth. In fact it is for the youth's emotional stability. The virgin promotes the moral and physical health of the community, and enters into marriage and sexual intimacy with self-confidence.

Secondly, let's discuss what appears in the Bible to be an equation of sexual desire with hunger, or a comparison between food and sex. In the New Testament era, some Christians at the church in Corinth seemed to have likened sexual desire to hunger. They, probably, reasoned that to have sex either within or without the marital union is to meet a need as natural and acceptable as to have a meal to satisfy hunger. But the Apostle Paul challenged that reasoning and equation. He argued that food is for the stomach, and the stomach has been designed for the assimilation of the food we eat. Every part of the body is designed for a specific and legitimate function. The body, generally, is not designed for sensuality. The human body has been designed for the glory of God, the Master-designer (1 Cor. 6:13, 20).

The equation of sexual desire with hunger is generally wrong. Hunger and sexual desire are two distinct phenomena. Their motivational factors are respectively, and distinctively, different. For example, hunger is a physical sensation that occurs when there is a lack of energy within the body. Energy is derived from food, and it is required for the proper function and maintenance of the body. Without the energy the body slows down and eventually burns out of function. On the other hand, sexual desire is externally stimulated. Unlike hunger it does not signal any internal lack or need which if not met would lead to a breakdown, causing physical harm and dysfunction of the entire body.

Sexual desire can and is controlled by shunning that which may externally draw the mind to lust after the flesh, and focusing the mind and thought on something that is eternally rewarding. After all, "Every man is tempted when he is drawn away of his own lust, and enticed" (James 1:14). Therefore, "Set your affection on things above, not on things on the earth" (Col. 3:2).

The Meaning of Human Sexuality

We trivialize human sexuality if and when we think of it as a means of procreation. Though it is, but God could have invented other means of human reproduction. We also cheapen human sexuality when we view it as a means of expressing pleasure. Sex is more than an act of meeting and satisfying a physical desire and need. There is more to sex and in sex than procreation and temporary sexual pleasure.

Human sexuality is a physical, emotional, and psychological expression of acceptance and belonging to each other for life. It is a sealing of a marital bond of knowing, sharing, and appreciating the unique characteristics of the man and woman. The body-to-body contact and touch experienced during sexual intercourse is symbolically a stamp of surrender of oneself to the other marital partner for a permanent and indissoluble marital relation. It is also an acknowledgement that the body of one sex partner exclusively belongs to the other sex partner in the marital relationship. Human sexuality is literally and physically knowing and entering the exclusively private chamber of your spouse, that which essentially and humanly differentiates the man from the woman. The male and the female are in their sexual intimacy physically and emotionally challenged to be true to each other, and to "keep their secret to themselves".

Furthermore, the biblical view of sexual immorality helps to understand the significance and meaning of human sexuality. The Bible indicates that to engage in illicit sex with another man's wife is to "uncover" the man's "skirt" (Deut. 22:30; 27:20, KJV). And to "uncover" the man's "skirt" means to expose his nakedness (Lev. 18:8; 20:11, 20, 21, KJV). What this connotes is that the man and the woman in marriage are exclusively a "covering" to each other.

The Moslem holy book, the Qur'an, re-echoes this biblical concept by its declaration that the spouses "are a garment" to each other (Sura 2:188; see also Sura 4:25).

A skirt or garment is a covering worn for protection or concealment. The "covering" is a pictorial representation of the physical, emotional, and spiritual warmth that the couple provides each other. Also in the picture is the confidential relationship between the man and the woman. Each is a confidant to the other, keeping the gender related secret that borders on their sexual peculiarities. By sexual intercourse each physically, emotionally, and psychologically "discovers" true and true the concealed "person" of the marital partner.

What they see, know, and experience sexually of each other becomes a "private" and confidential matter. In fact it is the sex organ and all that it stands for that becomes the couple's personal secret that should not be shared with anybody outside the marital union. Thus each spouse exclusively becomes a covering skirt or garment for the other.

The Biblical concept of human sexuality should be viewed from the setting of human reproductive organs. The external reproductive organ is the sum total of each sex. In other words, what a person is by sex or gender is embodied or epitomized in the person's reproductive organs. It should be noted that genital organs of the two sexes are designed to complement each other. For example, the genital organs of a male are activated and functional for an end only with contact of female genital organs. Importantly, too, the ideal domain of operation for the sex organs is exclusively within a marital union of male and female. Thus, an illicit sex distorts the moral significance and Biblical view of human sexuality. It makes a brute of womanhood and manhood.

The dignity or glory of humankind is degraded by directly or indirectly promoting sexual immorality, and unlawful or unconventional use of the sexual organs.

The meaning of human sexuality has been discussed in the context of heterosexual marriage. If we recognize and honor God's creation and established law, and if we believe that each part of human body is designed for specific function and use then homosexuality, anal intercourse, and oral-genital sexual activity are misleading and deviant sex expressions. There is one natural way of human sexuality, and only between man and woman. The sexual union involving penetration of the vagina by the penis is divinely and naturally established. To act otherwise is to make God look like stupid for his creation. As a matter of decency, fellatio and cunnilingus are bestial behavior that makes a lie to man's endowed dignity over and above all other creation on earth.

Warped Lifestyle

Warping mind or warping lifestyle?
One frowns, and the other smiles
At a he or she that mates with a same-sex
Population rusts and civilization rots
The "Homo" from hetero-sexual marriage
sees homosexuality alternative lifestyle
and outsourced heterosexual marriage to the Wild
for a scrambled lifestyle and a warped morality
See! Homosexuality exists on the strength and
dynamism of heterosexual marriage
Not a single "Homo" is born from a homosexual relationship
Making homosexuality absurd alternative, and
a warped lifestyle from a warped mind

Summary

We outline the major points and arguments of the work to better help us see and understand the issue and what is at stake with a lifestyle of cosmetics and a negative reaction to human complexion

1. The use of cosmetics for personal adornment is universal. Among the ancient people of Egypt, in particular, their idols were adorned with makeup. Perhaps to confirm their religious and cultural belief that social life and interaction continues somewhere at death.

2. Many hold the view that human complexions evolved millions of years past to meet varied climatic conditions on earth. But the Christian Bible indicates, however, those human complexions are a design and creation of God. The complexions are genetically determined and inherited from the first humans on earth.

3. The various skin colors of the human race are common features with other creatures. The Bible attests a common source for all the human color groups. Science, too, uncovers the inter-relatedness of chemical makeup of all the human skin colors.

4. The human skin colors are put in place not to divide mankind into races but to awaken in man the feeling and sense of an awesome Creator-God.

5. Immortal bodies with unchanging complexions await the redeemed at the coming of Jesus. Death and resurrection will not change any skin color.

6. Discontent with our complexion or an aversion for any human skin color and language group may be the result of childhood upbringing, social pressure, and personal choice. But biases, prejudices, and all acts of hate towards any one are downright disregard and rejection of God's explicit injunction to love all and hate no one.

7. Objections to the makeup are based on the implications and assumptions behind its use. Man is a vessel and temple of God. He is declared a perfect product of God's handiwork. Therefore, the use of makeup faults any claim to a perfect, wholesome creation. It is a discontentment with God's choice for man.

8. Cosmetics elicit attention and attraction to the self. Besides, preoccupation with outward appearance and beauty robs God of man's worship time, admiration and adoration due Him. And also robs man of God's time and opportunity to live a life that would attract men and women to his Creator.

9. Motivations for the use of makeup vary among its users. But all the motivations are characterized by self-centeredness, self-gratification, and self-glorification.

Conclusion

The world of fashion has glamorized the use of makeup, and has presented it as an indispensable part of modern life. Thus, many men and women, young and old, have turned to a painting spree of the eyelashes, eyebrows, nails, and lips. Every Christian should be aware that the word of God has warned against the use of any part of the human body for that which encourages and/or leads to sin. And when God's word requires man to offer the parts of his/her body to God "as instruments of righteousness" (Rom. 6:13), every sincere believer in the word of God should wonder how the paintings of those parts of the body would honor God. No one should assume that God's word, which is given through the Apostle Paul to all believers, is not to be literally interpreted to condemn the use of *makeup and manicure preparations*.[1]

Besides, no Christian should deny the fact that the Bible stands out clearly to condemn outward adornment. It recom-

---

1   Cosmetic preparations for improving appearance, among other things, with colorings, and/or bleaching materials. These include rouge, lipstick, eye/brow/lash/lid colorings; nail enamel, bleaching creams and etc.

mends, instead, humility, the unfading beauty of inner self, as of great worth in God's sight (1 Pet. 3:3, 4).

What is your motivation for wearing makeup? Is it to improve or enhance your physical appearance? My advice is simple: Be what you are the natural you. Cease wearing a mask. The pep and glamour of life finds their enduring expression and meaning in a decent and simple living. Is it worth the time and money to put on that which may corrupt the mind, and serve as a stumbling block to seekers of the truth, even when your conscience is clear and your motive is right? The limitation placed on your liberty (1 Cor. 8:9–12), should be considered as you make a choice between wearing the makeup beauty and the natural "you". The word of God calls for a transformation of the heart, and not a conformity to the lifestyle, custom and standard of the worldly. Count the hours that is spent before mirrors to improve the physical and external appearance with makeup. Could those hours have been spent on bended knees with a pledge before the throne of God: "Not I but Christ be seen and be known"?

A makeup lifestyle is a life lived for the self. It is a rejection of God's perfect work in man, and thus, a breach in inter-personal relationship with God.

In reality man is born for tomorrow. He has a future. There seems to be something special and natural in the morrow that motivates man to dream, think and plan for tomorrow. One of the characteristics of man as human is a feeling and sense of a better tomorrow. This also sets him apart from the beast. We are under an obligation to sit back and reflect upon the ultimate goal for what we put into life, in terms of our lifestyle as it relates to our human body, and in terms of our view and treatment of human skin colors.

Suffice it to say that a peaceful, death-free endless tomorrow is prepared for today. And it is not an outcome for a life lived unto the self here and now.

The Apostle Paul warns, "Be very careful how you live because the days are evil" (Eph. 5:15, 16). This is a call to reflect on the present in reference to the future. Life should be lived now in preparation for the future. We must make the best use of our time and life in preparation for the rough ride tomorrow. We must be wise to know that living at ease today cannot prepare us to face the turbulent wind of tomorrow. We must earnestly pursue that which can stand through both calm and rough times. The one and only thing that could follow us through life to the grave and beyond the grave is character. When the evil day comes we will naturally prefer safety to seeking artificial beauty. On that day the money and time spent to beautify the external and physical appearance to the neglect of the inner self will be a costly and unprofitable investment.

The concern for the "here-and-now" existence is sown like a seed into the fertile soil of the conscious and subconscious minds of our children when they are taught that the external physical and makeup look is indispensable for the survival of every woman.

Every Christian woman and/or mother must accept the fact that womanhood is neither a showcase for materialism nor a creation of fashion and makeup. It is not to the credit of either womanhood or manhood to be treated like a fattening cow and seen as a purveyor of sex. Flamboyant life that displays self and physical beauty is misplacement of values and trifling with the functional meaning of womanhood and manhood.

The Biblical portrait of true womanhood is noteworthy (see Prov. 31:10–31). By creation every woman is designed and equipped to bear and transmit life. Therefore, womanhood is basically and essentially a responsibility to build and preserve life. Womanhood subscribes to industry and frugality as a way of life. Womanhood values and works with time to minister to the basic needs of her family. Womanhood is not self-centered but people-centered ministry. Womanhood is not a movement for body and physical evolution but a power for moral purity. By divine purpose and appointment true womanhood shuns that which corrupts and marginalizes character.

Womanhood is not synonymous with hedonism, but a concern for fidelity. Womanhood is not a personification of deceptive charm and fleeting beauty, but a personification of a moral institution that abhors and wages war against corrupting influences of our time.

Womanhood is not a concern for external appearance to the neglect of the inward beauty.

It is, functionally, a responsibility to build character. In fact womanhood connotes partnership with God for preservation of life in its original beauty. It is by mutual law of partnership a rejection of all that would distort the handiwork of God.

Likewise manhood shares with all the virtues of true womanhood. In addition manhood is neither a display of physical prowess nor a promotion of physical charm. By divine appointment manhood connotes leadership. And leadership is follower ship in all that is real, pure and edifying. Manhood is not gender identity with muscle training but a gender role for character building. Manhood is not a developmental stage of physical maturity, but a developmental stage of responsible lifestyle that glorifies or honors the One in whose hands our breath is. Generally, manhood or womanhood is the ultimate developmental stage in humankind. It is characterized by mental, physical, and moral maturity, and reflected in authentic lifestyle that recognizes human body as God's temple. The grave responsibility of manhood and womanhood to live real and above superficial life leads to the contention that it is not worth the expense and time to decorate and beautify the skin only to be consumed by the flames at cremation, or be eaten up by the worms and decay at death. It is not fashionable to "skin" the body through bleaching for a change of color. It is unchristian to "tone" the skin when the heart is tainted with discontentment and self-centeredness.

Consider the fact that all of God's creations, from animate beings to inanimate objects, and from man to the minerals of the ground or rocks, are of varied colors. The minerals such as the opal, a solid crystalline chemical compound found in igneous and sedimentary rocks and the tourmaline are in black, white, blue, yellow, green, and red varieties. Men and women seek after these minerals of various colors today, as gems and jewels of immense value. It is foolhardy to seek after these minerals while man created in the image and likeness of God is treated with contempt for his skin color, and/or language group. Common sense teaches that what a person is by color is meaningful only in reference to others with similar and differing color.

Consider, also, by a contrast with a related problem, the misconception about human body. A mock advertisement written for a high school newsletter that was never published reads: "Wanted a medical breakthrough in harnessing human growth hormones to increase and/or adjust the height of dwarfs and giants of the world. The former with too little supply of growth hormone, and the latter with over-supply of it. Both needs medical attention. The situation is critical and challenging to medical science."

In contrast with skin color, dwarfism and giantism are both abnormal condition that will be normalized only by the Creator God in the earth made new. But none of the human skin colors is abnormal or defective skin condition. Therefore human body whatever its complexion should be off limit to the goddess of beauty.

Besides, the limitation of medical science to change one skin color into another is not puzzling. Because human body is not man's creation that could be manipulated at his discretion. We may call it freedom of choice to "improve" our skin for beauty, but in matters of beauty and eternity, it is not the end but God who determines and justifies the means to a beautiful end.

We noted earlier that hate crime may be motivated out of contempt for an ethnic or language group. It is argued that such contempt or hate is misplaced. Biblical account of the development of human languages points to God as the originator of every language.

Reflecting upon the factors that led to the birth of numerous languages and the abuses and misuses of these languages are a mental exercise that leads to some conclusions. One of the conclusions is an assertion that none of the languages, vehicles that carry and transmit our culture of hate and contempt is fit for adoption as a living and universal language for a recreated world. All the evils that are associated with or linked to human skin colors and languages, namely, racism, tribalism, sectionalism, and all the isms of divisiveness will not rear their ugly heads in the new world of love.

One of the realities of human life is that nothing is permanent on the planet earth. We should not fail to comprehend the fact that it is not what one enjoys today but what one will fail to enjoy tomorrow that would be of greatest concern for every rational being.

It is not what one may claim to be here and now but what one will fail to be hereafter is the crux of human existence. The word of God affirms: *"No eye has seen, no ear has heard, no mind has conceived what God has prepared for those who love him"* (1 Cor. 2:9; Isa. 64:4). Of course the ear of faith has heard the coming reality of eternal life declared in the word of God. The eye of faith has perceived the coming reality of immortal body for the redeemed of God. But our sinful nature here and now is a limitation to full comprehension of the breadth and depth of the coming reality.

However, it is satisfying hearing Prophet Isaiah echoing with prophetic utterances God's best to be restored back to those who love him. It is re-assuring listening to Apostle Paul re-echoing it with the zeal of a convinced and convicted believer in the second advent of Jesus. Men and women who are indeed convinced of a better world of God's making should live for the real and shun the artificial. They should know that wearing the face of Christianity with the heart and spirit of the world does much harm to the cause of God. After all, the word of God intimates that outwardly beautiful person without discretion is a reproach to beauty. But a foresighted person is a paragon of beauty (see Prov. 11:22). Beauty is personified in the one who looks beyond the present and immediate, and whose character draws someone to the Creator. Beauty is immortalized in something that outlasts this present life, endures through the here-and-now into the hereafter. That something is character.

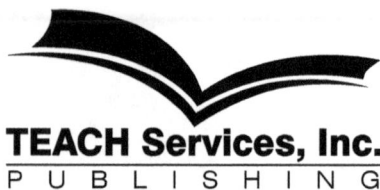

www.ingramcontent.com/pod-product-compliance
Lightning Source LLC
Chambersburg PA
CBHW060440090426
42733CB00011B/2343